# Dedic

To my Creator– The One from who all blessings flow.
Thank you for saving me, for turning my chronic illness into
my testimony of Your faithfulness, and for the passion and
excitement I get every time I share with others what you have
taught me.

For my husband, and my best friend, Jason Mauldin.
Thank you for choosing me, for supporting me through
chronic illness, for believing that we should follow the dreams
that God placed in our hearts, and for making those dreams a
reality.      You are truly one in a million!

# What people are saying about Vibrant Health...

*"I have been over weight for many years...By the time I reached 356 pounds I was taking 17 pills a day for High Blood Pressure, High Cholesterol, High Triglycerides, Diabetes, Asthma, Edema and Gout...I have spent a life time on every diet known to man...My wife and I signed up [for the Vibrant Health Course] and each and every week we would try one or two things from all the different things we heard. Almost instantly I really started feeling better, with a lot more energy and zest. The weight loss was steady...After two months I went to my doctor for a check up. I had quit taking a few of my pills as my Edema and Gout were no longer issues. I told him of my desire to get off all my medication. He was impressed with the 60 pounds I had dropped, but a week later when he got the results back from my blood work I don't think he could believe the results. Every number was in the normal range – something that has not happened for the 31 years I have been on the medications...The Vibrant Health class really helped a lot... it is more about eating the way GOD intended us to...I feel better and have more energy that I have had in twenty years."*

~R.T. Douglasville, Georgia

*"I have been implementing small things... well I have lost 5 pounds! I don't exercise nearly as much as I use to (1 hour of jog-ging  a day). I do 30-45 minutes of <u>walking</u> and I am still losing... Wow, I feel so blessed that you all have appeared in my life and blessed me and my family with this awesome gift of living healthy."*

~S. Sutton, Douglasville, Georgia

# VIBRANT
# HEALTH

SIMPLE STEPS TO TRANSFORM YOUR HEALTH

## BECKY MAULDIN N.D.

This book belongs to:

_____

**Vibrant Health:** Simple Steps to Transform Your Health
Copyright © 2011 by Becky Mauldin, N.D.
Pure Vitality
www.getpurevitality.com

Book Design and Layout by Becky Mauldin
Printed in the U.S.A.

# Table of Contents

# Introduction

Vibrant health is available to each and every one of us. Your body has the power to heal. You can be as healthy as you want to be. Our Creator designed our bodies to work perfectly. He created the human body with the inherent ability to heal. Think of a cut, or a broken bone. Given time, the cut heals and the bone mends. When the human body is given what it needs to function optimally, the body has an amazing ability to be healthy. That is vibrant health!

Many books on health are either overwhelming or overly-complicated to someone who is trying to become healthy. My goal is to simplify becoming healthy, to help you understand why healthy food is important, and to provide you with the tools that will enable you to make lasting changes in your own life. This book is a step-by-step guide to incorporating healthier foods into your life. All the recipes in this cookbook are not only easy to prepare, but they are delicious. I believe that food that is good for you must taste delicious!

Diet programs are focused on short term deprivation rather than building long term health. This book is not about dieting or restricting calories. This information is based on the solid nutritional research of Dr. Weston Price, Bernard Jensen Ph. D., and my experience. Their research has shown what our bodies need to be healthy.

Some people will use this material to take their health to the next level. Others will use this information to regain their health and reverse disease. But everyone will gain a better understanding of their body and the relationship food plays in our everyday health.

You will find that becoming healthier can change your life in ways that go far beyond just feeling better. Many times, people find that when they feel better or lose weight, they become open to trying new things or have the energy to fulfill their dreams and passions. Becoming healthier could be the catalyst that enables you to live life to the fullest!

# My Story

Up until my mid 20's, I had numerous common health issues: constipation, acne, PMS, mood swings, depression, canker sores, frequent indigestion, and low energy. I thought it was normal to have these issues all the time. I didn't know it was even possible to be free of these annoying health problems. When my mother-in-law was diagnosed with breast cancer, I started to look into the role that nutrition played in health. The more I researched, the more it just made sense to me. So, I used myself as a guinea pig for my own personal experiment. First, I began to clean up my diet, eliminating the sugar and processed foods. Amazingly, my health concerns started to go away. Second, I added more raw foods to my diet, and my health soared beyond what I thought possible. It didn't happen overnight, but once I started feeling the difference with better nutrition, I became committed to a healthy lifestyle. I simply couldn't believe that it was possible to wake up every day feeling great!

Years later, I was exposed to some toxic chemicals, and my health started to break down. Although I had been eating a healthy diet for many years, it suddenly could not reverse the damage being caused by the chemicals. Insomnia, fatigue, depression, thyroid problems, and adrenal problems robbed by of my energy and vitality. As my body became more and more toxic, my symptoms intensified. The constant headache, severe insomnia, and depression grew worse until I ended up with Multiple Chemical Sensitivity, which is a condition in which the body reacts to man-made chemicals and artificial fragrances.

This illness affected my life and family in ways that I could not have imagined. I had to run an air purifier at all times in my home. I could not go to the mall without feeling sick for days. I felt worse from the pesticides on grocery store produce. If I bought new clothes, they had to be washed a minimum of 5 times before I could wear them without reacting to the chemicals and dyes used in the manufacturing process.

I could no longer be around paints or do the hobbies I loved. Any new item from the store had to be washed or left outside to off-gas the new chemical smell, or it would cause me to feel terrible.

My health rapidly deteriorated in spite of my good diet and the supplements I was taking. I realized there was a piece of my health puzzle I was missing: detoxification. But I had no idea how to do that. I finally came to the point of surrendering my situation to God and trusting that He would provide the answer.

Three days later, a friend called to tell me about a practitioner she had just met that does sauna detoxification programs. It became crystal clear that this was the answer to my prayers, and I began a detoxification program at a clinic that utilizes a far-infrared sauna to remove the toxic chemicals from the body.

As I detoxified, my symptoms and allergic reactions began to go away. After several months of cleansing, I was regaining my health. Through this experience, I learned that I had been exposed to chemicals that were causing my body to break down. Mainstream medicine could not help me because pharmaceutical drugs are chemicals that would have only made me sicker. Because of my toxic body burden, my body was basically poisoned. It didn't matter how many good nutrients I consumed, because those toxins had to be removed before I could get better.

Through my experience and working with clients, I have learned that lasting health is only possible through a healthy diet and regular detoxification. I am now free of insomnia, adrenal and thyroid problems, chemical sensitivities, depression, and fatigue. I believe in the power of food and detoxification to heal the body and create vibrant health. So, whether your health problems are big or small, I've been there, and I can show you how to achieve vibrant health. So, let's get started!

# Gluten

Each and every recipe in this book is gluten-free. What is gluten? Gluten is the protein found in wheat, rye, barley, and some oats. Gluten is what makes bread dough so elastic and rise so easily.

## What's the problem with gluten?

For those with celiac disease, gluten causes the lining of the small intestine to be destroyed. This causes malabsorption and therefore, a host of health problems.

Other people have gluten intolerance. Similar to celiac disease, the immune system of the gluten sensitive person reacts when gluten is ingested. The gluten protein is attacked by the immune system as a toxin. This can result in extensive damage to the body, creating symptoms that affect digestion, mood, heart, liver, thyroid, reproduction, brain function, muscles and joints. For me personally, I get depression, acne, canker sores, and PMS from eating gluten. So I am highly motivated to avoid it!

Gluten intolerance is extremely common, affecting conservatively 20% of our population. Yet only 5% of the millions suffering know that their health problems are caused by gluten. Until recently gluten sensitivity was questioned as a condition. But it is now clear that it is a very valid condition affecting a great number of individuals.

Grains or flours that are free of gluten include rice, quinoa, buckwheat, millet, amaranth, sorghum, tapioca, nut flours, arrowroot, corn, and flax.

# What is optimal health?

Optimal health can be defined as experiencing the fullness of life **physically, mentally, and emotionally**. Health is much more than the absence of disease. Health is a state of vibrant well-being! But let's face it. Most of us don't even know what optimal health is. We are living in the most unhealthy society that has ever existed. People are willing to accept feeling just okay, and they expect to be tired and to have "normal" signs of aging. However, this is not normal! Just because it is common these days, does not make it normal.

**The traits of optimal health are:**
- A feeling of energy throughout the day
- A youthful appearance
- Sleep comes easily and you awaken refreshed
- You have no pain anywhere
- Skin is clear and smooth, with a pink glow
- Hair has a glossiness and shine
- The mind is clear and alert
- There is good posture with good muscle tone and flexibility
- A comfortable weight is maintained
- The eyes are bright, alert, and clear
- Teeth are bright white and well-aligned
- There is a cheerful disposition and stable emotions
- There is a good appetite and digestion
- There is a feeling of gratitude
- Obstacles and setbacks are seen as opportunities for growth
- There is a sense of purpose in life

The way to optimal health is not a secret. However, you are not going to learn about vibrant health in the mainstream media, and you are not going to learn about it from your doctor. It's not going to come from a pill, injection, or medical procedure. There are natural laws that govern our universe and when those laws are followed, they produce vibrant health. When these laws are broken, the result is disease.

What natural laws are we talking about?  How do these laws create vibrant health?  What do people who have vibrant health look like?  To answer these questions, we need to look at the research of Dr. Weston Price.

Dr. Price was a dentist in Cleveland, Ohio in the 1930's.  He began noticing that the children of his patients were having many problems he had not seen before: crowded, crooked teeth, rampant cavities, frequent infections, allergies, and behavioral problems.  He did not believe that this was God's plan for mankind.  His quest for the answer to these problems led him to travel the world for 10 years in search of people without these problems.

His travels led him to the corners of the earth where people were living without contact with modern civilization.  What Dr. Price found amazed him.  In 14 different isolated cultures, he found that tooth decay was rare or non-existent!  These people had never even seen a dentist or brushed their teeth!  He found that they were free from diseases, such as cancer, heart disease, tuberculosis, allergies, and infections.  Even the way they looked displayed their vibrant health—They had excellent bone structure.  Their faces were wide and well formed.  They had high cheekbones, and a broad jaw with beautiful, perfectly straight teeth, including their wisdom teeth.  They also had a broad pelvis that enabled the women to give birth with ease.  Their babies had no birth defects and were very robust and healthy.

When Dr. Price analyzed the food they ate, he found that it contained four times the minerals and 10 times the vitamins as the modern American diet of his time.  So, what did they eat?  Each culture ate different foods, depending on what they had available in their area.  In Switzerland, the people lived on raw milk and raw cheese, rye bread, meat, and fresh vegetables.  In Scotland, they ate fish, along with whole oats and vegetables.  In other parts of the world, hunter-gatherers consumed game animals, and a wide variety of grains, tubers, vegetables, and fruits in their area.

Each culture had one thing in common:  they ate foods in their natural form, just as nature provided them.  Their meat was from healthy animals on lush pastures, their fish came from the ocean, and their milk was raw, not heat-treated or homogenized.  They ate fresh fruits and vegetables, nuts, seeds, and whole grains.  By eating the foods that Nature had provided, they obtained all the nutrients needed by the body for it to be in perfect health.  These nutrients enabled them to have freedom from disease, cavities, and other health problems.

Weston Price found that in nearby, more modernized areas, where stores or outposts had been established, the native foods had been replaced by foods of modern civilization: sugar, white flour, canned goods, jams, pastries, and preserved foods.  He noticed that when the healthy people ate this food instead of their natural diet, they became sick, began getting cavities, and other diseases.  The children born to parents eating these foods had a higher incidence of birth defects and other problems that Dr. Price had seen in his practice: crowded, crooked teeth, poor bone structure, allergies, and infections.  These modern foods were not providing sufficient nutrients to allow the body to develop and to function as it was designed.  Because they were not getting enough vitamins and minerals, the children's bone structure had not been able to fully develop, leading to narrow jawbones without enough room for all their teeth, narrowed nostrils that created a tendency for allergies, and narrowed hip bones that caused difficult childbirths.  They were unable to reach their full genetic potential or attain vibrant health.

When Dr. Price came back to his office, he did an experiment with some of the malnourished children in his practice.  These children were eating mostly refined foods: coffee with sugar, white bread, pan-cakes, donuts, etc... Dr. Price fed these children one meal a day of nutri ent dense whole foods, while they still ate the same foods at home. He fed them rich meat stews with vegetables, fish, whole raw milk, and whole grain bread with butter. The children's health and performance in school improved markedly. The added nutrients in the whole foods Dr. Price provided enabled them to gain better health.

Weston Price stated that, "Life in all it's fullness, is Mother Nature obeyed." Nature is perfect in it's design, and has provided everything we need to be in optimal health. This is the natural law that we must live by. Weston Price documented the results of living according to Nature's laws, by eating nutrient-dense natural foods, and the results of going against those laws by eating man-made, nutrient-deficient foods. The consequences are astounding.

The human body was created to work perfectly. The quality of your health and well-being is not just left up to chance or fate. Nature has given us the perfect foods and if we eat according to what Nature provides, we will be healthy. But if we do not, our bodies were created with a 'warning system' to alert us to our bodies needs. Because the body is a self-repairing mechanism, it can heal itself. When it cannot heal, it will send out warning signs to us to alert us to the need for assistance. These signals are called *symptoms*.

Many of us don't pay attention to these symptoms we experience on a daily basis. In this culture, we are bombarded daily by advertisements for products designed to mask these symptoms, and rather than find the root cause of them, we have come to believe that the symptoms are "normal," and that they need to be suppressed. But if we only temporarily relieve the symptom and don't address the root cause, then it *will* escalate and cause further disease in the body. Each symptom is the way that your body is trying to alert you that something is wrong in your diet or lifestyle.

## Some examples of warning signs (symptoms):

- Bloating
- Gas
- Abdominal pain
- Low back pain
- Varicose veins
- Water retention
- Bad breath
- Ear infections
- Sore throat
- Soft or brittle nails
- Sensitivity to perfumes/ chemicals
- Insomnia or poor sleep patterns
- Brain fog
- Depression
- Mood swings
- Painful joints
- Fatigue
- Headaches
- Body aches and pains
- Acne, eczema, or skin rashes
- Angina
- Diarrhea and/or constipation
- Pain of any kind
- Shortness of breath
- Sensitive teeth/ gums
- Short attention span
- Dizziness
- Nausea

Symptoms are like the red light that flashes on the dash board of your car. There are 2 things you can do: Cover it up so you don't see it, or figure out what the car needs and fix it. Covering it up is like using drugs: They mask the symptoms and the damage to your body continues to get worse down the road.

A symptom such as pain is one way for the body to get our attention. To have pain and then to take a pain reliever so it will go away, is like covering up the light on the dashboard of the car so you won't notice it anymore. If you keep driving, you can easily ruin your engine, but if you stop and look under the hood, you could prevent a major problem down the road. Everyday, people drive their bodies without paying any attention to the warning signals. Pain relievers do nothing to relieve the source of the pain- they just hide the body's warnings. When people find themselves in a hospital with a health crisis, they wonder how it happened. The body was not taken care of and it eventually manifested disease.

*Disease does not just happen.* It is created. It is created when we ignore those little warning signs and do not give our body the necessary support it needs. We need to respect symptoms and see them for what they are: unhealthy lifestyle indicators. The best way to eliminate symptoms is to address the underlying cause and change what is wrong in your life. This is how natural healing works. Drugs only manage symptoms, and usually end up exchanging one set of symptoms for another due to their side effects. But natural healing corrects the problem that caused the symptoms in the first place.

When our bodies are operating on poor nutrition from processed foods, you can get caught in a cycle....you don't feel good, your energy is low, so you sit around all day, finding it hard to get up and take better care of yourself. You settle for junk food or processed food because it seems convenient, but it only perpetuates this cycle. When you understand what junk food is doing to your body on a cellular level, you see that your lack of energy and weight gain is actually happening because your body is malnourished and burdened with toxins, not just because you lack willpower. *You are altering your body chemistry with your food.* Understanding this can help empower you to change. Exercising more or going on a cleanse without first supporting the body with high quality nutrition is like asking the body to do more work with less fuel. It doesn't work very well. And you won't feel very good.

Therefore, the foundation for good health must begin with food. Understanding the body's need for high quality nutrition can help empower you to change what you eat. But that change must begin in the mind. Unhealthy habits have to be broken for change to happen.

The truth is: You have the power to change the way you feel. Your body has the capacity to rejuvenate. You can wake up every day feeling great with plenty of energy! As soon as you begin to feed your body well and take care of yourself, you will start changing your body chemistry for the better. Your body will begin to respond, and your level of vitality will increase as you start to experience more vibrant health.

What you eat and how you live has brought you to exactly where you are right now. If you keep doing what you have been doing, you are going to keep getting what you have been getting. The choices you have made yesterday do not have to have an effect on the choices you make today. Every day is a new day. Every day a new opportunity for change. Make the decision to change your life!

Change is not easy. But YOU are worth it! I don't know about you, but I was just sick and tired of being sick and tired. Once I started eating better and feeling better, I got addicted to feeling good! Are you ready for a change?

# The Problem with Processed Foods

Most Americans spend 90% of their grocery bill on processed foods.  Processed foods are made using modern methods and techniques that transform natural foods into another form by the food processing industry.  This generation of children is growing up on diets of mostly processed foods.  Many of them do not even *recognize* real food anymore.

Processed food did not even exist until recently.  Let's go back one hundred years.  What did people eat 100 years ago?  Was it natural?  Was it organic?  At that time, processed foods simply did not exist!  All food was natural.  And it was certainly organic since pesticides have only been in existence for the last 75 years.  Organic or natural foods are certainly not fads.  They are not some *new* thing.  If anything is a radical new thing, it is processed foods.

One hundred years ago, cancer accounted for only three percent of all deaths.  Now cancer causes 30% of all deaths.  That is one in three people!  The incidence of diabetes has risen from .1% in the year 1900 to more than 20% in the year 2011.  Heart disease was actually unheard of at the turn of the century and now it kills more than 700,000 people a year.  Autism did not even exist before 1929, the same year vaccines were developed.  In just the past few decades, the autism rate has gone from 1 in 2,500 children to 1 in 95 children.  Rates of disease are skyrocketing!  What has changed?  Our food.

What humans eat as food has undergone more profound change in the past century than in all the previous centuries.  Yet, we have the same nutritional needs as our ancestors.  This discrepancy between the food that Nature provides for us and what we now eat has created the current epidemic of chronic disease.

What has happened to our food?  Man has taken what Nature has provided and has decided to "improve" upon it.  We have taken natural foods and put them through processes that would preserve them practically forever, guaranteeing a long shelf life and more profit.  We think we have created something to solve our problems.  But have we really?

In the late 1800's, wheat began being refined by steel roller mills that were capable of stripping away the bran and the germ from the pure starch.  This process is what created pure white flour.  Companies wanted it because it would last longer than whole wheat flour.  However, as the use of white flour became more common, illnesses due to vitamin deficiencies began to appear.  The reason was because when whole wheat is refined into white flour, the amount of nutrients lost are extraordinary: 95% of the fiber is lost, 84% of the iron, 95% of the Vitamin E, 82% of the Manganese, 60% of the Calcium, 85% of the Magnesium, 78%, of the Zinc, 80% of the Niacin, and 81% of the other B Vitamins. In an attempt to compensate for these nutrient losses due to the manufacturing process, food processors  resorted to enriching the flour with just a few of the vitamins that were lost in the processing: some of the B vitamins and iron.  But the enriched flour is still missing up to 80% of it's nutrients! As Bernard Jensen says, enrichment sounds like such a nice term, but if a thief stole your car and left you with a bicycle, would you consider yourself enriched?

The problem is that those lost nutrients are necessary for proper human nutrition.  Research has found that most heart attack patients lack chromium, selenium and vitamin E.  Research animals become sterile when manganese is taken out of their diets.  Selenium is necessary for proper function of the liver and the immune system.  Pantothentic acid is used to produce hormones.  Vitamin A is vital for good vision and clear skin.  Niacin is needed for good digestion and calm nerves.  Vitamin E is essential for the heart and reproductive system.  Whole grains contain the proper balance of all these elements,  when they are left in their natural state.   The majority of these essential vitamins and minerals are absent from "enriched" bread.

Sugar is another food created by the food manufacturing industry. Sugar comes from the sugar cane plant. Eaten in its natural form the way traditional cultures consumed it, it did not cause dental decay. However, when sugar is processed, it has been stripped of the minerals and fiber leaving just the pure, white sugar. The missing nutrients- the B vitamins, magnesium, and chromium- actually help to maintain healthy blood sugar. When you eat refined sugar, your body gets a feeling of quick energy, yet it is denied the natural combination of nutrients present in the natural sugar cane that would keep it in balance. In order to compensate for the lack of nutrients, your body has to dip into your own reserves to help you metabolize the sugar. Instead of supplying nourishment, the refined sugar actually *robs* your body of minerals and vitamins. Minerals are taken from the body and used to neutralize the acidic effect that sugar has on the body. So much calcium is taken from the bones and teeth that decay and general weakening of the body begins.

Sugar also has a profound effect on the immune system. It suppresses the immune system for up to 5 hours after you eat it. Sugar has been linked to many other health conditions including cancer, heart disease, high cholesterol, fatigue, kidney stones, arthritis, depression, allergies, obesity, PMS, tooth decay, hormonal imbalances, diabetes, and hypoglycemia. Did you know that one can of soft drink contains an average of 10 teaspoons of sugar? Drinking one can per day will add up to 15 extra pounds of extra body weight per year, and many people drink even more than that.

Artificial sweeteners that contain aspartame are even worse for you than sugar. Aspartame was discovered by accident in 1965 when James Schlatter was testing an anti-ulcer drug, and it is now in over 6,000 different products. There are 90 different documented symptoms associated with aspartame and some of them are headaches, migraines, dizziness, seizures, numbness, muscle spasms, weight gain, rashes, depression, fatigue, anxiety, memory loss, joint pain, and breathing difficulties. In fact, this *one* food additive has accounted for over 75% of all the adverse reactions to food additives reported to the FDA. It is poison!

In an American Cancer Society study of 78,000 women, those who ate foods with artificial sweeteners actually gained *more* weight over a year than those who consumed foods sweetened with sugar! Artificial sweeteners are more of a hazard to your health than refined sugar.

Meat has undergone HUGE changes in the past 50 years. Up until the 1930's, most cattle were raised on green pastures, eating what Nature designed them to eat: grass. But now, cattle are raised in enormous feedlots that can hold up to one hundred thousand head of cattle. There is no longer any grass where they live. Instead they are fed massive amounts of grains along with waste products from poultry plants. This fattens the cattle quickly, along with steroids that are implanted in their ear. Because of the cramped space and high amount of manure, these cattle are prone to all sorts of illnesses and many of them harbor E.coli and other pathogens. Because of this, they are given antibiotics to cover up the problems, rather than correcting the underlying issue. Fortunately, grass-fed meat from healthy animals is becoming increasingly available from many stores and farms.

Monosodium glutamate, or MSG, is flavor-enhancing chemical that started being added to processed foods after WWII and the amount added to foods has doubled every decade since then. MSG belongs to a category of food additives called excitotoxins. MSG revs up brain amino acids that make one feel "up", stimulated, or slightly excited, leading to addictive eating patterns and obesity.

Dr. Russell Blaylock stumbled onto this research when he found that his own children were so hooked on a particular brand of canned spaghetti that they craved it for every meal. He found it was the MSG that provoked the craving reaction in the children. As he researched this food additive, he was startled to find that MSG wears out the nerves through hyper-stimulation. MSG and similar food additives can destroy the nerve cells, specifically in the inner layers of the retina and in an area of the brain that controls the glandular functions of the body. He found that as little as a single dose of MSG can trigger nerve deterioration. It is added to many processed foods to enhance their taste. MSG can be found in most broths or bouillion, spice mixes and seasonings, Chinese food, soy sauce, soups, salt substitutes, some salad dressings, steak sauces, lunch meats, and any foods with hydrolyzed proteins or yeast extract.

Fats and oils are another food that has been harmed by industrial food processing. Most oils are now extracted in factories using high heat and pressure which damages the oils and weakens the carbon bonds of the fats. When they are subjected to high heat, the oils can become oxidized or rancid. These rancid oils cause free radical damage in the body. Free radicals are unpaired electrons that are extremely chemically reactive in our bodies. They attack cell membranes and red blood cells, damage our DNA, and damage organs and tissues, setting the stage for tumors and the buildup of plaque in the arteries. Studies have shown a high corrolation between cancer and heart disease with the increasing consumption of these highly processed oils, such as canola oil, soy oil, and vegetable oil.

Margarine or tub spreads are made from hydrogenated oils. Hydrogenation is a process that turns oils that are liquid at room temperature into fats that are solid at room temperature. For this process, manufacturers use the cheapest oils (soy, corn, or canola) and mix them with tiny metal particles, usually nickel. Then it is subjected to hydrogen gas in a high-pressure, high-temperature reactor. Next, soap-like emulsifiers and starch are added to the mixture to give it a better consistency. The oil is then steam cleaned at high temperatures to remove the unpleasant odor. Dyes and artificial flavorings are then added to make it resemble butter. These partially hydrogenated margarines and shortenings are even worse for you than the highly refined oils they are made from because of the chemical changes that occur during the processing. These changes produce the most dangerous fats: Trans fats. Trans fats have been linked to cancer, heart disease, immune system breakdown, depression, fatigue, and hormonal imbalances. 90% of all processed foods contain these hydrogenated or partially hydrogenated oils.

The body is designed to take in high quality nutrition and convert it to usable energy. Natural foods are able to supply the necessary nutrients for good health and growth. But when foods are processed, many nutrients are removed or destroyed in the manufacturing process. These foods do not have enough of what our bodies need: vitamins, minerals, nutrients, and enzymes. These missing nutrients are what the body uses to build new cells and tissues, and to carry out it's functions. Processed foods satisfy hunger by providing calories, but with little nutritional value. When we have an excess of calories with very few nutrients, the calories are stored as fat and degenerative diseases will soon follow.

When the body is given natural foods that contain all their nutritional factors, the body knows exactly when it has had enough to eat and it will shut off the appetite just as abruptly as one would shut off a water faucet. But when processed foods are eaten, it throws off this balance and the body keeps looking for the nutrients that normally go along with the calories. The appetite is increased in an effort to get the important vitamins, minerals, and enzymes it is lacking. This is the underlying cause of cravings. Junk foods and processed foods that are missing nutrients cause us to keep eating, and eating, and eating, because our body is looking for the vitamins and minerals it is *not* getting.

Processed foods are also loaded with chemicals and preservatives. The problem with these chemicals is that our bodies were not created to utilize them. *Our bodies see these chemicals as invaders or toxins.* Therefore, your body must use your liver to detoxify these chemicals and render them harmless to you. By eating processed foods, you are increasing the toxins in your body. When your body is exposed to more chemicals than it can successfully detoxify, the body will then store the chemicals in your fat cells. In the detoxification process, the body uses antioxidants to neutralize the free radicals produced by these manmade chemicals. Your body's main antioxidant is called glutathione.

Your cells use glutathione to create energy and to keep you healthy. However, it is used up when our body has to detoxify the harmful chemicals and preservatives we are exposed to. When your glutathione levels drop, your body's ability to create energy drops, causing fatigue. These toxins cause cellular inflammation, which leads to the degeneration of your body. When in the inflammation in your heart, you can have heart attacks or heart disease. When it is in your pancreas, it can cause diabetes. When it is in the brain, it can cause Alzheimer's disease. Cellular inflammation can lead to every disease known to man.

Here is the key point you need to remember: Natural foods are recognizable by the body and can assimilated, whereas unnatural food-like substances are toxic to your body and will actually contribute to the degeneration of your organs, weight gain, and premature aging.

This means you will never again have to look at anything other than the ingredients in a product to know whether or not it is good for your body. If it has white flour, sugar, high fructose corn syrup, hydrogenated oils, or chemicals you can't pronounce in it, it is not fit for human consumption.

So, what happens when you eat processed food? While natural foods are able to move through the digestive tract easily and quickly, processed foods are hard for the body to break down, and they stay in your digestive tract for a long time using up a large amount of energy in digestion, leaving you feeling less vibrant. What happens over a lifetime of eating processed, hard-to-digest foods? A major backlog develops, turning a healthy digestive tract into an unhealthy system where bad bacteria can thrive and your elimination slows down. This leads straight to constipation, obesity, and many degenerative conditions. Poor digestion and the excess waste matter that your body is not able to eliminate efficiently is at the root of many health problems.

When you eat nutrient-dense, whole foods, you will begin to notice an increase in your energy level and less of a desire for sugar and other non-nutritious foods. Because you are getting all the nutrients you need, you will need less food to fill you up and satisfy you. If you are overweight you will find that it will be easier to lose weight eating nutrient-dense foods. And if you are underweight, your weight will normalize.

Food is not just fuel for your body, it is also the building material for your body. What you eat today is going to be part of your memory, part of your bones, your teeth, your hair, and your heart tomorrow. The reality is: YOU ARE WHAT YOU EAT.

Are you comfortable with your current level of health? Good health is something that is easy to take for granted. We are not motivated to do anything about it, until disease strikes. Then we shift our priorities and make it important. Don't wait for disease to strike. Don't wait for those minor health concerns to turn into bigger ones. Make your health a priority now, so that you will have good health in the future. The truth is that without good health, you cannot enjoy life.

# It's Your Decision

Before you move on to the next section, I want you to evaluate where you are and decide if you are willing to change by taking some baby steps in the right direction. Are you ready to make your health a priority? Are you ready to start feeling better?

Fill out the **Health Inventory Form** and the **Motivation to Change** on the next few pages if you are ready to take that step. This information will help you keep track of the beneficial changes you will experience in your health as you start on this amazing journey. A few months from now, this form will help you see how far you have come and will inspire you to continue on the path to vibrant health!

# Health and Food Intake Inventory

Name:_____        Date:_____

Please list your main health concerns in order of importance:
1. _____
2. _____
3. _____
4. _____

Current weight:_____   Blood pressure:_____   Blood sugar:_____

Current symptoms:  (check all that apply and explain)
☐   Energy: 1 (low) - 5 (high):_____
☐   Sleep (how many hours and quality):_____
☐   Mental /Mood:_____
☐   Skin:_____
☐   Digestion:_____
☐   Elimination (how often are your bowel movements?):_____
☐   Pain level:_____
☐   Allergies (food or environmental):_____
☐   Male/Female organs:_____
☐   Respiratory system:_____
☐   Immune system:_____
☐   Stress level:_____
Physical activity (type and how often):_____

## Food Intake (list everything eaten past 24 hours)

Breakfast:_____   Time:_____
Lunch:_____   Time:_____
Snacks:_____   Time:_____
Dinner:_____   Time:_____
Water intake:_____
Beverages:_____
Medications or supplements:_____

_____

# Your Motivation to Change

Identifying the reasons for wanting to change your diet is very important for helping you to achieve your goal. This will help you to support yourself during this process.

What was the main thing that made you want to start eating a healthier diet? (The answer usually involves a moment when you realized that something in your life was not the way you wanted it.)

_____
_____
_____

What are 3 specific obstacles you see that could hinder your success?
1. _____
_____
2. _____
_____
3. _____
_____

What are some strategies you can use to overcome obstacle #1? What are some things that you can do to help you with this?

_____
_____

What are some strategies you can use to overcome obstacle #2? What are some things that you can do to help you overcome this?

_____
_____

What are some strategies you can use to overcome obstacle #3? What can you do to help you overcome this?

_____
_____

**Example:** Obstacle #1: _I get hungry when I'm out and eat fast food._
- New strategies: _I keep healthy snacks, such as nuts or bars in my purse or car in case I get hungry. And, I schedule my outings after I have already eaten a meal._

List a few health goals you are interested in achieving:

1. _____

2. _____

3. _____

How will you feel when you reach these goals?

_____

_____

What will you be able to do once you achieve these goals that you do not feel capable of doing now? _____

_____

_____

Identify images, words, songs, etc…that can help you achieve your goals.

- Find pictures or images that will remind you of your goals and place in prominent locations to keep you motivated.  Post an image or picture of what you will look or feel like.

- Find words or phrases that you can have friends and family say to you when you need encouragement.

- Tell your family and friends specific ways they can support you. Invite a friend or family member to make changes with you.

How will you celebrate your success? (It could be a party, new clothes, a trip, or something else that is meaningful to you.) _____

_____

Who will you invite to celebrate with you? _____

_____

This section was adapted from *Great Cleanse Lifestyle Journal* by Dana Kuebler N.D.

# Myths & Truths About Food

In this section, we are going to talk about some specific myths that you may believe about food. These are statements that you have heard in the media or from advertisements. When you hear these statements repeated often enough, eventually you begin to think it is the truth. But you will see that many of them are just myths that have been created to benefit the industrial food system.

**Myth #1:** *Heart disease is caused by cholesterol and saturated fats from animal foods.* Heart disease was non-existent before the early 1900's. The first heart attack was documented around 1906. This is when people were living on farms, eating meat, butter, eggs, and whole milk. Food had not yet begun to be processed and so these foods were full fat products. These were animals who were eating grass, not grain. During the period of rapid increase in heart disease, from 1920- 1960, the consumption of animal fats actually declined, while the consumption of hydrogenated and processed vegetable oils increased dramatically. It is clearly not the animal fats that caused heart disease. If butter and animal fats caused heart disease, it would not be a new disease. The truth is, a study in the 1994 edition of the Lancet medical journal found that the fatty acids that have been clogging arteries are mostly unsaturated fats. It is the vegetable oils!  In Nutrition Week from March 22, 1991, a study shows that people who eat margarine have twice the rate of heart disease as those who eat butter.

When you examine the animal fats, the meat of pasture raised animals has less fat than the meat of animals fed exclusively grain. The fat of grass eaters has a beneficial nutrient called CLA, which stands for conjugated linoleic acid. This is a fatty acid which studies indicate may help reduce weight, protect against heart disease and prevent cancer. Feedlot animals eating only grain, have no CLA in their fat. So, you can see that even nutritionally, there is a big difference between grain fed and grass fed animals.

**Myth #2:** *Animal foods are not healthy so the only way to be healthy is to be a vegan.* A vegan is someone who eats NO animal foods of any type. No meat, no dairy, no eggs, and no fish. The truth is that mankind has eaten animal foods since the beginning of time. In fact, when you look at history, there has never been a culture that has only eaten plant foods. Weston Price did not find any truly vegan cultures in the 14 different cultures he studied. In his travels across the globe, all of the cultures included some form of animal protein in their diets. And if we look back into time even beyond Weston Price, *all* cultures in the history of the world have eaten animal foods. Every single one. Whether it was raw milk from pastured animals, meat from wild game, seafood, or insects, they all consumed some form of animal products. When you look at the cultures who had the highest rates of longevity, they all consumed animal products. Traditional animal foods are not to blame for our increasing rates of disease.

Human beings are omnivores. Our digestive tract is neither short like a carnivore, nor very long like an herbivore. Ours is somewhere in between. Our teeth are made up of flat molars designed to chew vegetables and sharp teeth designed to eat meat. Omnivores can eat all foods, both animal meat and plant foods.

It is only recently, that the vegan movement has taken hold, and people are abstaining entirely from animal products. But problems are arising from this. Many modern day, long-term vegans are finding that they are becoming deficient in certain vitamins that can only be found in animal foods, such as B-12, Vitamin A, Vitamin D, EPA and DHA. Some vegans have even gotten permanent neurological damage from a lack of B-12 in their diet. Because of that, many prominent leaders in the vegan movement are encouraging vegans to take a B-12 supplement. What this should be telling us, is that humans were not designed to be vegans. Veganism is not healthy if it results in a B-12 deficiency. Lindsay Allen, the director of the U.S. Human Nutrition Research Center, says that "when women avoid *all* animal foods, their babies are born small, they grow very slowly, and they are developmentally retarded." She goes on to say, "There's no question that it's unethical for parents to bring up their children as strict vegans."

Many Americans **over-consume** animal protein and do find **tremendous** health improvements when they cut out the animal protein for a short period of time. A vegan diet is an excellent *short-term* diet to cleanse and heal the body, especially if raw fruits and vegetables are the bulk of the diet. But if you choose to eat that way long term, I would encourage you to listen to your body and be open to the possibility of eating naturally-raised animal products occasionally to maintain your health.

**Myth #3:** *To be healthy you need to eat a low-fat diet.* The real problem is not the fats. The problem is that people tend to eat the wrong kinds of fats: fats that are highly refined and processed. Fats are important to our health. Without adequate fat, vitamins A, D, E, and K could not be absorbed into our bloodstream to nourish our body. Fats also are used for energy. The membrane of each one of our cells is made of fats. Fats enhance immune function, protect us from cardiovascular disease, and support healthy hormonal balance. Natural fats such as butter, extra virgin olive oil, coconut oil, cold-pressed sunflower, cold-pressed avocado, sesame and flax oil are fats that have nourished people for thousands of years. Natural cold-pressed oils are easily metabolized by the body and do not contribute to weight gain like the highly refined oils.

Low fat or no fat diets can actually be dangerous to our well being. A study in the Lancet found that low fat diets are actually associated with increased rates of depression, psychological problems, fatigue, and violence. Children on low-fat diets suffer from growth problems, failure to thrive, and learning disabilities. The proper fats are vital to our health. Low-fat products are loaded with additives, sugars, and preservatives to make them taste better, but are even worse for your body than the fat they removed. Stick to natural whole foods and the natural fats your body needs.

**Myth #4: *Soy is good for you.*** Food processors have created more soy products than ever before: soy milk, soy cheese, soy yogurt, soy burgers, etc... Many people are switching to soy because they think it is healthier. The truth is that modern soy foods do not provide the same health benefits as traditionally prepared soy. Cultures that consumed soy regularly always fermented it. The natural fermenting process breaks down the phytic acid and enzyme inhibitors, which can inhibit the assimilation of minerals and cause digestive problems. Many modern soy foods are not fermented and are processed in a way that denatures the proteins. Non-fermented soy foods can cause low thyroid function, infertility, and mineral deficiencies. Highly processed soy foods also result in high levels of free glutamic acid, a potent neurotoxin. In infants, the consumption of soy formula has been linked to autoimmune thyroid disease. Soy milk, soy cheese, soy yogurt, and other meat substitutes made from soy, are highly processed and are best avoided. Soy foods are healthiest eaten in their traditional fermented form, such as in tofu, tempeh, natto, miso, and tamari.

**Myth #5: *It is too expensive to eat natural food.*** When we look at the percentage of income that Americans spend on food, it is only a fraction of our total income. It is only about 9%. That is less than any other industrialized nation spends on food! Thirty years ago, it was a good bit higher: 15%. If we look at other countries around the world, you will find that Americans spend less than any other country on food. Germans spend around 11% of their income, Japan is 13.4%, South Korea is 13.4%, France is 13.6%, South Africa is 17.5%, Mexico is 21%, and China is 28%. This shows us that in general, many Americans really *could* afford to allocate more of their income to food. Many of us can come up with the money to pay for the latest new technology, so is this really a matter of affordability or priority?

There is a misconception that natural foods cost more, but when you look deeper, you will realize that the price of the food is not on the price tag. When you buy processed foods you pay an additional cost for the packaging, the marketing, and the preservatives. There are additional costs added for the processing, storage, shipping, distribution, and retailer profit. A fraction of the price you pay is for the food itself. When you buy processed foods, you essentially pay double - one time for what is in the package and then again for the adverse effects it has on the body. Money saved foolishly today will be spent many times over on doctor's bills tomorrow.

Another way to look at it is, if you were to take the money that you normally spend on prescription drugs and medical expenses, and buy nutrient dense foods, you may find that you may not need to *go* to the doctor or *take* drugs anymore! Spending more on food can help you reduce your medical expenses.

Even if you just don't have the financial resources to spend on food, there are ways to get good quality food. Growing your own vegetables is one of the best ways to save money. A few dollars worth of seeds can yield many pounds of produce. Another way to save money is to buy food in bulk. You can buy grains, like rice and oats, beans and lentils in large quantities from food co-ops or farmer's markets at a discount, and they will provide many nourishing meals. Another idea is to find a local farm in your area and see if they would like some help. Several years ago, I volunteered at a local organic farm for a few hours each week in exchange for 2 huge grocery sacks of produce! It can be a win-win situation for both you and the farmer.

**Myth #6:** *If I exercise regularly and take supplements, I don't need to be as concerned about what I eat.* Because we are used to the Western medical model, in which a pill is taken for a symptom, we tend to think the same thing applies to natural health. In our culture, we think that if a headache is "cured" by an aspirin, then our other health problems should be "cured" by a vitamin supplement. We do not want to address our diet or our bad habits. But vibrant health does not come from a pill, or even a natural supplement. As I have already discussed, it ultimately comes from food.

In order to achieve vibrant health, there are very specific steps that you need to follow. They need to be done in this order:

1. **Healthy Food and Clean Water**
2. **Exercise**
3. **Nutritional  Supplements**
4. **Detoxification**

The first place to start is your food and water intake. Nutrient-dense food provides the *foundation* for a healthy body. Just as a good foundation is necessary for a well-built house, so it is with the body. If your foundation is not strong, I don't care what else you try to do to get well. It will not work.

Next, you need to address any bad habits that are not conducive to health and start exercising regularly. Poor sleep, lack of exercise, smoking, drinking alcohol, a stressful job or relationship, or exposure to toxic chemicals are continual stressors that inhibit the body's ability to regenerate and repair itself. These things, just like a poor diet, can set the stage for illness to gain a foothold and keep you from achieving vibrant health.

The third step is to take nutritional supplements. Nutritional supplements can help make sure all your nutritional needs are being met. While many people feel like we can get all of our nutrition from food, it is becoming increasingly difficult due to lowered soil fertility, shipping food long distances, food processing, and a lack of freshness. There are a few supplements that can really help take your health to the next level. I have included a basic list to get you started on page 80.

The last step on your journey to vibrant health is detoxification. Man-made pollution has ensured that everyone on this planet is now toxic. The Environmental Working Group found the umbilical cord blood of newborn babies contains over 200 man-made toxic compounds. These are people who have not even come into the world yet! Every one of us is now exposed to these chemicals and we need to take steps to minimize exposure and detoxify. There are several ways to do this, but using a far-infrared sauna on a regular basis is one of the best ways to remove these toxins from the body.

Colon cleansing is another very important way to detoxify the body. Because processed foods are hard for the body to break down, they stay in the digestive tract for a long time. What happens over a lifetime of eating processed, hard-to-digest foods? A major backlog develops, turning a healthy digestive tract into an unhealthy system where bad bacteria can thrive and your eliminative channels slow down. This leads straight to chronic constipation. Nothing in your body can be healthy if you are reab-sorbing toxic waste that was meant to be eliminated from your colon. We put so much effort into cleaning the outside of our bodies, but what about the inside? Our skin will never be healthy, our organs will never be healthy, our bloodstream will never be clean until the large intestine is clean and healthy. Every cell in your body becomes as toxic as the condition of the intestines because every cell is dependant upon the nourishment picked up in the intestinal tract.

These steps to vibrant health are important, but many people tend to invert the order of these steps by taking a natural pill for their ill, just like the modern medical model. But the natural health model does not work this way. If you are not eating good food, you are only going to get temporary relief of your problem. I've had some people say to me, "I've tried herbs and they just didn't work for me." They will not work very well if your diet is high in sugar and processed foods. Supplements are just that: supple-ments. They are meant to supplement your diet with specific nutritional factors, but they cannot make up for a poor diet.

Another common error many people make as they try to get health-ier is to start out with a cleanse or detox program without changing what they eat. Detoxification is important, but the problem is that you cannot successfully detoxify an undernourished body. That is like asking your body to do more work with less fuel. Your body will not eliminate the tox-ins effectively unless it has the nutrients to replace them with.

# Differences Between Natural vs. Medical

| | Natural Healing | Medical System |
|---|---|---|
| Symptoms: | Pay attention to symptoms. See symptoms as the way our body communicates what it needs. | Suppress symptoms. Never get to the root cause of why the symptoms are there. |
| Focus: | To create a healthy person. | To destroy, kill, or cure a disease. |
| Method of Treatment: | Remove obstacles to healing, so the body can heal itself. This is done through changes in diet, exercise, detoxification, and emotional healing. | Attacking, killing, and removing disease using drugs and surgery. |
| Therapeutic Products: | Products of Nature that have no side effects: food, herbs, natural supplements, etc.. | Man-made products with many side effects: pharmaceutical drugs. |
| Modalities: | Food programs, cleansing and detoxification, exercise, supplements, massage, emotional healing, etc... | Surgery, chemotherapy, radiation, drugs, etc... |
| Emotions: | Positive Attitude: trust, strength, empowerment | Negative Attitude: Fear, anxiety, being out of control, etc... |
| Responsibilities: | I take responsibility for my health. I am in control. | I "caught" this disease, so I am a victim. The Doctor must heal me. |

# The Keys to Vibrant Health

I want you to think of this book like a road map.  It will give you the general way to vibrant health.  But just like a map, there may be several roads that lead to the same destination.  Some people will find that they need to eat animal meat regularly.  Others may find a vegetarian diet suits their body better.  We are all different with unique backgrounds and individual body chemistry.  This plan will get you headed in the right direction on the road to vibrant health.  As you eat healthier, you will learn how to listen to your body and choose the foods that are most compatible with YOUR body.

Although there is not a one-size-fits-all diet for everyone, I *have* found that for the majority of people, there are certain key elements that will lead to vibrant health.

•**Vegetables**  The first element is a diet high in vegetables.  The current food pyramid tends to emphasize the foods that are high in carbohydrates.  The majority of your daily food intake should actually come from vegetables.  Why vegetables?  Because they are powerhouses of nutrition and naturally low in calories.  They contain Vitamin C, beta-carotene, folic acid, calcium, magnesium, fiber, and many more nutrients.  They also contain a wealth of phyto-nutrients.  These are what give the plant it's color.  Scientists are continuing to discover the health benefits of each one of them.  Loaded with antioxidants, vegetables also help to fight disease and the effects of aging.

You are probably thinking, "Vegetables?? I don't like vegetables."  Do you ever wonder why you do not like them?  Maybe it is because they do not taste good to you.  Maybe you never grew up eating vegetables.  Maybe you were forced to eat vegetables.  Whatever the reason, I want you to know that there are legitimate reasons for this.  One reason you may not like vegetables is because processed foods are loaded with artificial flavors, MSG, and other flavor enhancers that chemically stimulate your taste buds to want more of whatever you are eating.  Your taste buds get corrupted by sugar and the chemical flavorings. Of course, broccoli tastes bland compared to Doritos! Your taste buds think Doritos are a party in a bag! Once you stop eating artificially flavored foods, your taste buds will become accustomed to the flavors of natural foods. It takes about 6-8 weeks for your taste buds to change and acclimate to natural foods.

Another reason most people don't like vegetables is because of the poor quality of conventionally-grown produce. Have you ever had a warm, ripe, just-picked tomato from a garden? How would you compare the taste of that tomato to the cold, mealy ones in the supermarket that were shipped from another continent? The difference is night and day. And that difference can determine if you like vegetables or dislike them. Believe it or not, Nature designed fruits and vegetables to taste good. Man, in an effort to grow more food, faster and cheaper, has industrialized farming so that produce is grown in a very different way than Nature does. To locate a farm near you, see www.localharvest.com.

## The Vibrant Health Food Pyramid

The ratio of foods you eat should be: 6 vegetables daily, 2 fruits daily, 1 starch daily, and 1or 2 proteins daily. This proportion should keep your diet 80% alkaline foods and 20% acid forming foods. Most people on the typical American diet eat too much protein and way too many sweets and starches.

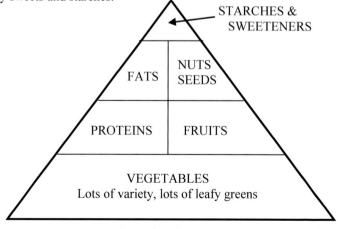

• **Organic** It is important to eat food free of pesticides & harmful chemicals. Pesticides are used to destroy insects by disrupting the nervous system of the bug, eventually killing it. Pesticides are poisons. They are meant to kill. While they do not kill us outright, some researchers believe that ingesting small amounts of them over a period of years can potentially lead to neurological problems, reproductive problems, lowered immunity, and chronic disease. Did you know that of the thousands of pesticides that are in use today, only a fraction of them are tested for their safety?

When food is grown without pesticides, herbicides, or genetically modified organisms, it is called, "organic." For many people, "organic" means "healthy." But you need to understand that organic simply describes one aspect of how the food was grown. It means that food was grown without pesticides or chemicals. It does not mean anything else. Some large processed food manufacturers have jumped on the organic bandwagon and are making packaged foods out of organic ingredients, and marketing them as healthier because they are 100% organic! You can even buy organic Pop Tarts and organic microwavable frozen dinners. Theoretically, even a Twinkie can be made from organic ingredients. But are these foods really good for us? Haven't they still gone through a lot of processing, which lowers nutrient content? How close are those foods to what is found in nature? Don't be fooled. Just because it says "organic" does not automatically make it healthy. As you start to increase your intake of raw fruits and vegetables, don't worry if they are not *all* organic at this point. Your goal is to get more real foods into your body. I would rather you eat non-organic apple, than an organic Pop Tart. In just a minute, you will understand why.

• **Raw Foods** Raw foods are fresh, living foods that have not been cooked or heated. Why raw foods? Because they contain enzymes. Enzymes are molecules that allows a chemical reaction to occur efficiently. Enzymes do many things, both inside our cells and outside our cells. They help provide energy to fuel our cells. Our immune cells use enzymes to attack and kill bacteria, viruses, and fungi, as well as dangerous cancer cells.  In the stomach, digestive enzymes, such as pepsin, are released by the lining of the digestive tract to help break down and digest the food we eat.

Not surprisingly, enzymes, as busy as they are, wear out and need to be replaced.  And as we age, our bodies' natural supply of enzymes becomes depleted.  The problem is that we are born with a limited supply of enzymes and they have to last us a lifetime.  When we eat a diet composed of processed, cooked foods, we will eventually begin to use our own enzyme reserves just to digest this type of food.  This places a *huge* burden on the body and makes us more susceptible to aging and disease.

Enzymes are only found in fresh, raw foods.  Temperatures above 115 degrees kill enzymes, and we cook our food at much higher temperatures than that!  Cooking destroys *all* of the enzymes in food. When you eat raw food, it has the enzymes in it that are necessary for it to be digested easily and efficiently.  When you eat cooked food, your body has to use it's own enzymes to digest the food, taking more energy from your body to accomplish this process.  Have you ever become sleepy after a big meal?  The reason is that your body's energy is being drained in order to digest the cooked food.  Processed foods, which are heated to even higher temperatures in the manufacturing process, are even harder for the body to digest.  This is one reason why people are drawn to coffee, caffeinated beverages, and sugary foods in an effort to increase their energy level when they eat mostly cooked foods.  When you eat raw foods, your body will start to feel more REAL energy then you could never get from a cup of coffee, because your body doesn't have to expend so much energy in digestion.

Raw foods also prevent constipation and weight gain.  Raw foods have a higher amount of vitamins, minerals, and enzymes than cooked foods.  While raw foods are very beneficial, you do not need to eat ONLY raw foods.  A diet made up of a high percentage of raw foods, such as 60%-80%, is one of the best ways to achieve vibrant health.

• **Green Juices**  Juicing fresh vegetables is another great way to get all the benefits that raw foods provide in bio-available form. A juicer separates the fiber from the juice of vegetables and fruits, leaving you with only the pure, natural juice.  Therefore, the juice is a concentrated source of vitamins, minerals, enzymes, and phyto-nutrients. Juicing is the best way to get the maximum amount of nutrition and enzymes from living foods without having to eat all of those vegetables to do it!  Fresh green juice can have a dramatic impact on health and well -being.

Juices are one of the most easily absorbed form of nutrition available.  Within 20 minutes of drinking fresh juice, the nutrients are already in your bloodstream and nourishing your cells.  They are absorbed without expending any digestive energy.  Because of that, juices can heal and rejuvenate the body quickly like no other food can. By removing the indigestible fiber from the vegetables, nutrients in the juice are more bio-available to the body than if the vegetables were eaten whole.

Fruit juices are not recommended for building health due to the high amount of natural sugars in the fruit.  It is the green color that is in vegetables that has been found to be most healing to the body. Chlorophyll is what makes plants green.  The chlorophyll molecule has been found to be almost identical to the human body's hemoglobin part of the red blood cell.  Many practitioners believe that chlorophyll-rich foods help to build the blood, increase oxygenation in the body, and provide the nutrients that reverse disease.  Green juices are also highly alkalizing to the body and help to create a more alkaline pH in the body that promotes health.  Cancer cells cannot survive in an alkaline environment.

Vegetable juices should be made from a base of mild-tasting, juicy vegetables, such as carrots, zucchini, squash, cucumber, spinach, parsley, and celery.  Stronger tasting vegetables can be juiced, but should be used in smaller amounts to maintain palatability.  These can be kale, dandelion greens, beets, sprouts, other leafy greens, wheatgrass, lettuce, etc... Apples, lemons, limes, and fresh ginger root can be used in combination with the vegetables to make the green juice more palatable. There are lots of tasty juice recipes on page 84. All of the vegetables and fruits used for juicing should be organic if possible to minimize pesticide exposure.

### • Foods that are Easy to Digest  The most healthful

foods for the body are the easiest foods to digest. Raw foods and fresh raw vegetable juices certainly meet this requirement.

Fermented foods, such as yogurt, kefir, kimchi, sauerkraut, have been pre-digested by lactobacillus bacteria and support healthy digestion by supplying beneficial enzymes to the body. Consuming fermented foods regularly helps prevent constipation and enhances digestion. It is excellent for people with weakened digestive systems, which is often the result of eating processed foods.

While many of the commercially available fermented foods are pasteurized, which destroys the enzymes and beneficial bacteria, it is easy to make your own fermented foods. Sauerkraut and kimchi are two examples of fermented vegetables that you can make at home from the recipe on page 123.

Homemade broth is another food that is very easy on the digestive system and provides numerous health benefits. Broth is made by simmering meat and bones in water, along with vegetables. There has been a decline in using the bones to make broth in this country. Now, people use canned broths or bouillion cubes which are loaded with neuro-toxic monosodium glutamate. But our grandmothers and ancestors knew the benefits of broth and made good use of the bones of animals and fish when they made it.

Meat and fish stocks are used almost universally in other traditional cuisines, but have almost completely disappeared from the American kitchen.  This is a shame because, as every chef knows, it is broth that makes soups and sauces taste so good.

When they are properly prepared, broth is extremely nutritious because it contains minerals from the bone and cartilage in a form that is easy to assimilate.  The most important health benefits com from the gelatin the broth contains.  Gelatin is very unique because it supplies hydrophilic, or water-loving, properties to the diet.  This means they attract liquids.  Gelatin attracts digestive juices to the surface of cooked foods and allows rapid and easy digestion.  Raw foods also contain these hydrophilic colloids, which is what makes them easy to digest.  When foods are cooked, they become hydrophobic, meaning they repel digestive juices.  This is another reason why cooked foods can be harder to digest.  However, because gelatin attracts liquids even after it has been cooked, it aids in digestion by attracting digestive juices to the surface of cooked foods, making them easy to digest.  That is one reason why homemade chicken soup is so good for you when you are sick.  Just a small amount of gelatin-rich broth added to your meals with cooked food will help facilitate easy and efficient digestion.

Gelatin-rich broth have been used therapeutically in the treatment of digestive and intestinal disorders, such as hyper-acidity, colitis, and Crohn's disease.  Gelatin has been used for anemia, ulcers, diabetes, muscular dystrophy, and even cancer.  Modern research has confirmed that broth helps prevent infectious disease.  The soluble components of cartilage and collagen in stock are beneficial to those with rheumatoid arthritis and other joint problems.

# How it works

This chart gives you a clear picture of what types of food are easy or hard for your body to break down and utilize.  Foods higher on the chart are high in nutrients and low in toxins.  Foods lower on the chart are low in nutrients and high in toxins.  Locate your current diet on the chart and types of food you eat in each column.  When you make changes to your diet by moving up in any combination of columns, you will take the burden off your digestive system, have more energy, and a higher level of health and vitality.  If you eat mostly processed foods, and make a change to mostly raw foods, you will notice a more dramatic improvement in your health.

**The goal to achieve more vibrant health is to gradually modify your diet so you are eating according to the <u>top 2 rows </u>of the chart:** mostly raw fruits and vegetables with some easily digested animal proteins, nuts, seeds, and fermented foods.

Look at the bottom row of the chart.  This is the type of food many Americans eat.  Highly processed, nutrient-deficient, loaded with pesticides and herbicides, and no enzymes.  Can you see how the typical American diet is more likely to lead to health problems and disease?  These foods are low in every category!!  These foods are not only deficient in nutrients, but they place a huge burden on the digestive system.  So, from looking at this chart, you will see why I said that I would rather you eat a non-organic apple than an "organic" Pop Tart.  The apple, although it is not organic, is at the very top of the chart in most columns:  While the Pop Tarts are all organic, they actually rank lower in other categories.  This means that they are not as nutritious and are going to be somewhat taxing on your digestive tract.  When you look at the food of healthy cultures around the globe, they consumed foods that would fall into the first two rows of this chart.  They ate foods that were fresh and raw, naturally fermented, and lightly cooked.

| | Type of food | Organic? | % of raw | % of Nutrients |
|---|---|---|---|---|
| **Easiest for the body to process** | Raw foods, raw juices, fermented foods | 100% organic or wildcaught | 80-100% raw | 100% of nutrients intact |
| | Lightly cooked foods, soups, eggs, fish, beans, poultry and natural meats | 80% organic 20% non-organic | 80% raw 20% cooked | 75% of nutrients intact |
| | Over-cooked foods, Processed meats, whole grains | 50% organic 50% non-organic | 50% raw 50% cooked | 50% of nutrients intact (many destroyed by heat) |
| | Non-fermented soy products, enriched flour, pasteurized dairy | 20% organic 80% non-organic | 20% raw 80% cooked | Many nutrients destroyed by processing |
| **Hardest for the body to process** | Junk food, candy processed foods, fried foods, imitation foods | Non-organic | 100% cooked | Most of nutrients destroyed by processing |

When I first changed my diet years ago, organic foods were extremely hard to find. In fact, I don't remember even knowing what organic foods were at first. I just ate more fresh fruits and vegetables and started cooking with natural foods. I slowly cut back on the processed food in cans and packages. I gave my taste buds time to readjust to real food and I grew to love it.

As you move up the chart, you will notice improvements in your overall health and wellbeing. You might notice that your energy level increases, your mind becomes more clear, and your emotions are more stable. In fact, I hope you get hooked on feeling great like I did! Nothing provides as much motivation to keep going as feeling great. And nothing provides that feeling better than alive, vibrant, nutrient-dense foods!

# Where to Start:  Baby Steps

Here is a step-by-step plan for easily implementing this information into your life without getting overwhelmed.  This plan is based on taking small baby steps.  It is not about making drastic changes.  You start with one small step at a time, incorporate it into your life, then move on to the next step.  As you continue to keep taking steps to add healthier food into your diet, you will transform your health!

**Baby Step 1:  Drink a Smoothie**   Smoothies are one of the easiest ways to get fresh, living, nutrient-dense foods into your diet.  With just one smoothie a day, you can get 5 or more servings of fruits and vegetables!  Start with one of the recipes on page 82 to get you started.

## Baby Step 2: Eat a Healthy Snack
Replace the sugary snacks or junk foods you have been eating with something fresh.  The easiest thing to do is to eat a piece of fruit and a handful of nuts, or trail mix.  Check out the Appetizers and Snacks chapter for other tasty ideas.

## Baby Step 3: Eat Regular Meals
Eating regularly will keep your metabolism high, keep your blood sugar and your weight stabilized.  And yes, that means you should be eating breakfast.

## Baby Step 4: Add Raw Vegetables to a Meal
The addition of a raw vegetable to a meal of cooked food will help supply extra enzymes and nutrients that will help you to digest your meal more easily, and will increase your overall intake of raw foods each day.

## Baby Step 5:  Switch to Healthier Foods
Replace what you normally eat with more natural alternatives.

## Baby Step 6:  Plan for Success
Use the recipes in this book, the shopping lists, and menu plans to establish a system that will make it easier for you to eat this way for life.

# Baby Step 1: Drink a Smoothie

Smoothies are the ultimate healthy fast food. They take only a few minutes to prepare and are loaded with nutrient-dense, raw foods. With just one smoothie each day, you will get 5 or more servings of fresh fruits and vegetables!

To make a smoothie, the only equipment you will need is a blender. You can also use a stick blender, which is convenient to use at work or on the road. You can just blend your smoothie right into the cup, rinse off the stick blender, and drink.

The main ingredient is ripe fruit, such as bananas, pears, peaches, mangos, berries, etc.. Then you can add some almond butter or whey powder for protein, rather than a highly processed protein powder. A natural sweetener, such as stevia or honey or even dried fruit is all the sweetener you will need. Throw in a small handful of fresh spinach leaves or other green leafy vegetables. Add any optional flavorings, such as vanilla extract, cinnamon, almond extract, etc... and enough filtered water, almond milk, or other liquid to cover the solid ingredients and blend until smooth.

When the bulk of the smoothie is fruit, it will taste sweet. You will not even be able to taste the leafy greens. Start out with a small amount- just a small handful of leaves. The greens are important because you will be getting more minerals and chlorophyll than if you just used fruit alone. If you do not have any fresh greens on hand, you could substitute a green superfood powder instead. Just start with a half teaspoon and you can work up to more over time.

Try the recipes on page 82 for some tasty smoothie recipes. Incorporate smoothies into your routine before moving on to the next step.
*Note: Fresh green vegetable juices can be substituted for the smoothies.

# Baby Step 2: Eat a Healthy Snack

Replace the sugary snacks or junk foods you have been eating with fresh raw food. The absolute easiest thing to do is to eat a piece of fruit and a handful of nuts, trail mix, or granola. At this point, I want you to cut out sugar from your diet as much as possible. Sugar is addictive, and can continue to cause cravings if you eat it regularly.

Fresh fruit, like an apple, comes perfectly packaged by Nature in a convenient, single-sized serving, kept fresh for days until the moment you bite into it. Apples are great because they will last the entire week without being refrigerated. And there are so many varieties of apples! Each one has their own distinctive flavor. Some of my favorites are Gala, Fuji, Braeburn, Golden Delicious, Cameo, and Pink Lady. Do not even bother buying Red Delicious. It was bred for color and shape, but has virtually no flavor. Learn to pick out a good apple: It should be firm with an even color, without soft spots. The key to ripeness is to look at the bottom. The red color should go all the way to the bottom of the apple. If there is a little bit or a lot of green at the bottom, it is not ripe. A good, ripe apple is worth seeking out!

Raw nuts or bars can be stashed in your purse or desk drawer at work for the ultimate in convenience. Larabar is one brand of a raw snack bar that you can keep with you in case hunger strikes. If you have extra time to prepare foods, you could fix one of the desserts from the book, such as the fruit Cobbler or Power Bars. I make a batch at the beginning of the week, and they last for a week if your family or co-workers don't find them!

If you are used to eating popcorn regularly as a snack, switch from the microwaved version with artificial flavorings to one you can make yourself with an air popper. Drizzled with some melted coconut oil and sea salt, it tastes *amazing*. When I serve it to people in my classes, they go nuts over it!

# Quick, High-Energy Snack Ideas

- Carrot sticks or red bell pepper slices with Hummus (page 96)
- Trail mix or granola
- Fresh fruit and raw nuts
- Homemade beef jerky
- Whole grain crackers and raw cheese or a spread
- Tortilla chips and salsa
- Smoothies made into popsicles
- Larabars or other natural bars
- Dates stuffed with cream cheese or coconut butter (page 179)
- Raw apples with Caramel Apple Dip (page 180)
- Plain yogurt (dairy or dairy free) with honey and fresh fruit
- Homemade popcorn
- Fruit leathers
- Muffins
- Homemade cookies with natural ingredients

# Baby Step 3: Eat Regular Meals

Skipping meals or going more than 4-5 hours without eating is an unhealthy habit and can have a major impact on your health. Your body needs a steady supply of fuel to function optimally.

Breakfast is one of the most important meals of the day. If you are not hungry for breakfast, you may want to eat a lighter dinner several hours before bedtime. Eating large meals late at night can cause the digestive system to be overburdened, leading to lack of hunger in the morning. Skipping breakfast can have a major impact on the rest of your day. Here's why: Blood sugar, or glucose, is the fuel for every cell in your body. So, of course, you want your fuel supply to be constant all day long. Eating meals at regular intervals throughout the day is necessary to maintain this balance. Breakfast is important because it lays the foundation for the rest of the day.

Typical breakfast foods, such as cereal, bagels, donuts, pancakes, waffles, and toast with jam, are all high in sugars and simple carbohydrates which cause the blood sugar to spike and then crash. When your blood sugar drops too low (after these type of foods or eating nothing at all) many symptoms can occur. The first symptoms to set in are usually mental difficulties because the brain requires a lot of fuel to do it's job. It also requires amino acids, which come from protein, not carbohydrates. So, you may have trouble concentrating, being forgetful, or mentally dull. For optimal mental performance, eat some protein with breakfast.

Keep healthy snacks, such as nuts or bars in your purse or car, in case you get hungry while you are busy, so you do not need to skip a meal or resort to unhealthy food.

# Baby Step 4: Add raw vegetables to a meal

I want you to add a raw vegetable side dish to a meal. It can be a salad. It can be something simple like carrot sticks, red bell pepper strips, or cucumber slices. It could be a serving of kimchi, which is a delicious mixture of garlic and ginger seasoned raw fermented vegetables. Or it can be more elaborate like the raw carrot soup, pesto-stuffed mushrooms, or another recipe from this book. You could add a raw sauce to go over your meat

The addition of a raw vegetable to a meal of cooked food will help supply extra enzymes that will help you to digest your meal more easily, and will increase your overall intake of raw foods each day. If you are already eating raw vegetables with your meals, then good for you! You can move on to the next step. This baby step is for people who are still eating mostly cooked food for lunch and dinner. This will help to slowly transition them to more raw foods.

The goal we are aiming for is for fruits and vegetables to make up the majority of your daily food intake. About 75% of the volume of food you eat should be vegetables and fruits. The remainder is made up of protein, starches, sweeteners, and fats. You should have one or two servings of protein per day, and one serving of grain or starch per day. This ratio is ideal for maintaining the proper pH of the body, which is necessary to be free of disease and illness.

The typical American diet is too high in protein, and too high in starches. The alkaline minerals from fruits and vegetables are missing, which creates an acidic environment in the body that is prone to disease. When your diet is acidic, you are more likely to get arthritis, heart disease, cancer, PMS, constipation, and many other health problems.

# Baby Step 5: Switch to Healthier Foods

Take a look at the processed foods you have been eating and start to switch to healthier alternatives. Look at your favorite foods and think about which ones may have a healthier version. For example, you may like popcorn. Then switch from the micro-waved version with artificial flavorings to one you make yourself on the stovetop with organic popcorn kernels, coconut oil, and sea salt. If you are not ready to give up cheese, then switch from the pasteurized version with additives to raw milk cheeses, which can be found at stores like Whole Foods. Start using whole grain bread instead of bread made from white flour. Replace candy bars with organic 70% chocolate bars. Start to replace commercial meats with more naturally raised meats without the antibiotics and hormones. Continue eating the healthy foods you have already been eating and look at the other foods you eat and try to find better choices. The chart on the next page will give you more specific information on what to replace certain foods with.

Just start with one or two things and slowly incorporate them into your life. By doing this, you will be getting more nutrient dense foods into your body, and less foods with harmful chemical additives and preservatives.

| INSTEAD OF THIS: | REPLACE IT WITH THIS: |
| --- | --- |
| Bread made with white flour | Whole grain breads |
| Boullion cubes or pastes | Homemade broth |
| Cereal with sugar | Oatmeal or other whole grains |
| Canned fruits and vegetables | Fresh or frozen fruits/vegetables |
| Candy | Dried fruit and nuts or raw bars |
| Cheese (processed) | Raw cheese |
| Cookies with sugar, hydrogenated oils, and preservatives | Cookies made with whole grains, natural sweeteners, and good fats |
| Deli meats with nitrites | Organic meats without nitrites |
| Eggs, commercial | Organic eggs from healthy hens |
| Fish, farm-raised (fed soy products) | Fish from the ocean (wild) |
| Ice cream with sugar | Coconut milk ice cream |
| Margarine or hydrogenated spreads | Organic butter or coconut oil |
| Mayonnaise with soy oil | Homemade or organic mayo |
| Meats, commercial with antibiotics | Organic or grass-fed meats |
| Milk, pasteurized/homogenized | Raw milk from healthy animals |
| Oils, highly refined soy or canola | Cold pressed natural oils |
| Pasta made with white flour | Pasta made with whole grains |
| Popcorn, microwaved | Popcorn made at home |
| Rice, white | Brown rice |
| Salt, iodized and refined | Sea salt |
| Soft drinks | Juices, teas, etc.. |
| Syrup with sugar or corn syrup | Maple syrup or Agave nectar |
| Tap water | Filtered water |
| Vinegar, white | Raw apple cider vinegar |
| White flour | Whole grain flour |
| White sugar | Honey, agave, stevia, molasses |
| Yogurt, sweetened with sugar | Organic yogurt with  no sugar |

# Foods to Enjoy ~75% or more of the time

- **Fruits**: fresh, frozen or dried without sulfites
- **Vegetables**: fresh or frozen (canned tomatoes are good)
- **Nuts and seeds**: raw (not roasted) or as nut butters
- **Meats**: organic or grass fed
- **Fish**: ocean-caught (not farmed)
- **Whole grains**, and 100% whole grain bread without preservatives (Ezekiel bread), gluten-free breads
- **Eggs**: organic or high omega-3
- **Dairy**: organic and raw is ideal, nut milks
- **Fats**: organic butter, cold-pressed olive oil, cold-pressed coconut oil, avocado oil, sunflower oil, sesame oil, lard (organic)
- **Sweeteners**: raw honey, agave nectar, stevia, organic maple syrup, Rapadura brand unrefined sugar in moderation
- **Beans and Legumes**: dried (soaked before cooking) or canned
- **Soy**: Fermented soy such as miso, tamari, tempeh, natto, tofu
- **Condiments**: Raw apple cider vinegar, organic mustard, organic ketchup, organic mayonnaise, herbs and spices (without additives), sea salt, flavoring extracts without sugar added (vanilla extract, etc…), salad dressings made with olive oil (not canola or soy), salsa
- **Beverages**: purified water, naturally sparkling water, herbal teas, fresh fruit or vegetable juices

# Foods to eat less often ~ 25% or less

- **Fruits**: canned with added sweeteners
- **Vegetables**: canned
- **Nuts and seeds**: roasted
- **Meats**: commercially raised with hormones and antibiotics
- **Fish:** farm-raised fish, and tuna fish (due to high mercury content)
- **Eggs**: commercially raised with antibiotics

- **Dairy**: pasteurized and homogenized commercial dairy products, non-organic dairy products
- **Fats:** Canola oil, peanut oil
- **Sweeteners:** heated honey, sugar alcohols (xylitol, sorbitol)
  **Condiments**: with added preservatives or sugar, seasoning mixes with additives or MSG, salad dressings with canola or soy oil and preservatives, refined salt, pasteurized vinegars
- **Beverages:** coffee, black tea, tap water, pasteurized juices, wine

# Foods to Avoid Completely

- **Meats**: highly processed meats or imitation meats (such as lunch meats or hot dogs with nitrites and preservatives)
- **Deep fried foods**
- **Eggs**: imitation eggs (such as Egg Beaters)
- **Dairy:** processed cheese (Velveeta), sweetened condensed milk, ultra pasteurized products, commercial ice cream, non-fat dairy products, soy milk and soy yogurt
- **Highly refined grains** (anything made with white flour: bread, rolls, crackers, cereals, pastry),
- **Commercial cereals** made from puffed or shaped grains or high in sugar and artificial flavors/colors
- **Fats:** soybean oil, corn oil, vegetable oil, margarine, hydrogenated tub spreads, shortening
- **Sweeteners**: artificial sweeteners (Equal, etc..), high fructose corn syrup, sugar, corn syrup
- **Beverages**: Diet and regular soft drinks, sports drinks with sugar and preservatives, hard liquor
- **Genetically modified foods:** corn, soy, etc..
- Any product with hydrolyzed soy protein, monosodium glutamate, artificial flavors, colors, or chemicals

# Baby Step 6:  Plan for Success

If you have already implemented the Baby Steps so far, you have already improved most of your diet!  This section will give you the resources to help you put it all together, and create an ongoing life-style of making meals that will nourish you as you continue this journey.

On the next few pages there is a 2-week menu plan and shopping lists to get you started.  You will notice that there are several servings of fruits and vegetables each day, a moderate amount of protein, and a fairly low amount of carbohydrates.  This is the most energizing way to eat for most people.  It is gluten-free (no wheat, rye, oats, or barley) and dairy-free because most people feel healthier when they eliminate wheat and dairy products from their diet.

This plan is set up so that you will not be spending all of your time in the kitchen.  You will shop for food one time per week.  Food preparation time can be tailored to your schedule.  If your weeks are busy, you can set aside a block of time on the weekend where you pre-pare several main dishes and side dishes to eat during the week.  Or you may find you have the time to prepare meals each day.  Either way you choose, this plan is set up for the working family who doesn't have as much time to put into food preparation.  Leftovers are strategically util-ized to make the following day's meals a breeze.

## Have a Routine

One of the most helpful ways to make it easier is to have a routine for most meals, so that you will not have to think about what you are going to eat each day for breakfast, lunch, and dinner.  By now, you probably already drink a smoothie for breakfast everyday.  If you have a salad, a sandwich, or leftovers for lunch, and fruit or nuts for a snack, then the only meal you will have to think about is dinner.  There is an example of a menu plan on the following pages that includes break-fast, lunch, snacks, and dinner. I do not expect you to write out your entire menu this way, but this is to show you what type of things to eat for each meal.

Looking at this you will see that you can eat the same type of thing for breakfast most mornings, and a salad, leftovers, or a sandwich for lunch. Dinner is really the only meal that I have to put any effort into. Although each meal is made from scratch, there is really very little time spent each day in the kitchen. Dinner usually takes no more than 30 minutes to cook each night. Some nights it is even quicker than that when I just thaw some leftover soup from the freezer.

I have created this 2-week menu plan, along with shopping lists, for you to start with using the recipes from the book. If you want to use your own recipes, then write down what you eat regularly and make your shopping list from it. The form on page 70-71 is perfect to use for that purpose. Make copies of it and write out your meals for the week and beside it write down what you need to buy. Cut off the shopping list and take it to the store with you and put the menu on your refrigerator.

## Stock Your Kitchen

In addition to this menu plan, I have included a list of Staples, which are basic ingredients that are good to always have on hand. When you have a well stocked kitchen, all the ingredients you need to put together a meal are at your fingertips. It becomes easy to put something together at the last minute if you need to. Whether you are a planner or a procrastinator, you will be prepared. You can follow your plan, or you can deviate according to what sounds good at the moment. When you keep certain staples on hand, you will be able to put together a variety of meals, even without a plan.

# Menu Ideas

When you keep a well-stocked kitchen (see next couple pages), basic ingredients can be used to create many of the meals in this book.

Here are some ideas for meals:

## Breakfast Ideas

- Smoothies
- Fresh fruit
- Oatmeal
- Muffins (whole-grain)
- Pancakes (whole-grain)
- Omelet or a fritatta
- Yogurt and fruit
- Eggs with sautéed vegetables
- Almond butter on bread or a bar
- Natural sausage and eggs

## Lunch Ideas

- Salad with lots of veggies and protein
- Sandwich or wrap with whole-grain bread, vegetables, and natural meats
- Homemade soup and a salad
- Leftovers from previous meals
- A large smoothie

## Dinner Ideas

- A meat (fish, chicken, etc..) and cooked vegetables and a salad
- Soup and a salad
- A one dish meal such as spaghetti, fajitas, or a stir fry with lots of vegetables
- A large salad and a baked potato or sweet potato
- Anything from the breakfast section
- Hummus and an assortment of fresh vegetables and some bread

## Snack Ideas

- Apple or other fruit and nuts
- Apple slices and almond butter
- Trail mix
- Popcorn (homemade)
- Tortilla chips and salsa
- Raw fruit cobbler or pie
- Hummus and veggie sticks
- Whole grain crackers with hummus or raw cheese
- Yogurt and fresh fruit

# Tips for Making it Easy

- **Make food according to your schedule.** Food preparation can be shortened each day by setting aside one day each week to prepare several dishes for the upcoming week. You can make 2-3 different main dishes, 3-4 vegetable side dishes or salads, and a grain. You have created your own convenience foods that you can rotate through during the week. Just reheat in a toaster oven (not the microwave!) oven, or stovetop and serve. It does require a 4-5 hour block of time to cook and prepare the foods, but it can make the rest of the week a breeze.

- **Freeze food.** When you make soups or stews, doubling the recipe can provide leftovers that can be frozen in individual size containers for quick easy meals. Keep your freezer stocked for those times when you don't want to cook. Pancakes, waffles, or muffins can be made in larger quantities and frozen. Just warm them up in a toaster oven.

- **Make larger quantities.** When you cook grains or beans, it is more time efficient to cook a large quantity to have on hand to use in various ways throughout the week.

- **Make the most of your food.** If you make a roast chicken for dinner one night, be sure to save the leftover bones/carcass to use for making broth. Use it the next day or freeze it for another time. If you take off the remaining meat from the roast chicken and save the bones, the meat can be used during the week for many different meals: in chicken salad, in soups, in stir-fries or sautéed dishes, fajitas, quesadillas, etc... The broth can be used to make soups, stews, braises, and to cook grains.

- **Create new habits.** Remember that changing your menu will take effort initially, once you get into the habit of making new dishes, it becomes much easier.

# Ingredients: Staples to have on hand

## Pantry Staples:

Raw apple cider vinegar

Soy Sauce

Cold-pressed Olive oil

Coconut oil

Brown rice and other grains

Raw nuts and seeds

Beans, canned and dried

Lentils, dried

Organic tomatoes

Organic nut butter

Raw honey, agave, or stevia

Organic condiments

Avocado or sunflower oil

Sea salt

Balsamic vinegar

Organic popcorn

Gluten-free pasta

Coconut milk or butter

Organic maple syrup

Flax seeds

Dried fruit, unsulfured

Sun-dried tomatoes

Organic herbs and spices

Vanilla extract

Baking soda

Baking powder

Snacks: tortilla chips, granola bars, raw food bars, trail mix, etc.

## Meat and Dairy Staples:

Organic meats

Organic cheeses

Organic eggs

Organic butter

Wild-caught seafood

Plain yogurt

Uncured lunch meats

Milk (rice or almond milk)

## Produce Staples:

Onions

Garlic

Carrots

Celery

Lemons

Lettuce greens or spinach

Other vegetables that you prefer

Apples and other fruit

Frozen berries

# Kitchen Equipment

**Saucepans and a sauté pan**  Stainless steel, enamel coated cast iron, or glass is recommend over non-stick or aluminum cookware.

**Stockpot**  A large upright stockpot will enable you to save time by making a gallon or more of stock at a time.

**Blender**  A high-speed blender, such as a Vitamix, is nice for making smoothies, sauces, and other recipes from this book.  If you don't use a Vitamix, Oster makes a nice blender.

**Food processor**  Cuisinart makes a nice, dependable food processor.

**Colander**

**Knives**

**Roasting or Broiling pan**

**Baking dishes**

**Mixing bowls**

**Cutting Board**

**Measuring Cups and Spoons**

**Baking Sheets**

**Juicer**  This is optional, but highly recommended.  I've used many juicers over the years, but the Jack La Lanne Power Juicer is my favorite because it is easy to clean and takes up less space on my counter.

**Coffee grinder**  A small coffee grinder that is not used for coffee is very handy for grinding up flax seeds, nuts, and herbs in small quantities.

**Dehydrator**  This is optional.  If you want to eat a bigger variety of raw foods, dehydrated foods can be very helpful.  The Excalibur is the brand I use at home and recommend.

# Week 1 Menu Plan

| | Breakfast | Lunch | Dinner |
|---|---|---|---|
| **Mon** | Banana Nut smoothie<br><br>Snack: apple and cashews | Spinach salad with hard boiled eggs, avocado, onion, walnuts, and a vinaigrette | Roast chicken with roasted vegetables and potatoes |
| **Tue** | Mango Smoothie<br><br><br>Snack: Popcorn | Leftover chicken on mixed greens and vinaigrette | Raw Marinara |
| **Wed** | Fresh fruit salad and nuts<br><br>Snack: Trail mix and an apple | Sandwich on whole grain bread with leftover chicken, lettuce, sprouts, and avocado | Fajitas with guacamole and salsa, served on lettuce instead of in a tortilla. |
| **Thu** | Blueberry and Banana Smoothie<br><br>Snack: Raw bar and some fruit | Leftover fajita salad topped with guacamole and salsa | Raw Vegetable Chili |
| **Fri** | Almond butter on toast and fresh fruit<br><br>Snack: apple and cashews | Hummus with vegetables and crackers | Broiled salmon, steamed broccoli, and fresh sliced tomatoes |
| **Sat** | Banana Nut Smoothie<br><br>Snack: Yogurt and berries | Leftover salmon on salad greens and chopped vegetables | Turkey burgers, sautéed onions and mushrooms with spinach, and baked sweet potatoes |
| **Sun** | Fritatta<br><br><br>Snack: apple and trail mix | Leftover turkey burgers or Hummus and vegetables | Broiled fish, zucchini and onions, peas |

# Shopping List for Week 1

## Produce:

- ☐ Bananas: 1 bunch
- ☐ Mango: 2
- ☐ Apples: 4
- ☐ Berries: 1 lb
- ☐ Spinach: 1 bag
- ☐ Avocados: 3-4 ripe
- ☐ Red Onion: 1
- ☐ Lettuce: 1 container
- ☐ Yellow onion: 1 bag
- ☐ Carrots: 1 lb. bag
- ☐ New Potatoes: 1 lb.
- ☐ Tomatoes: 4 large
- ☐ Garlic: 1 head
- ☐ Parsley: 1 bunch
- ☐ Zucchini: 6
- ☐ Lime: 1
- ☐ Bell peppers: 3
- ☐ Green onions: 1 bunch
- ☐ Portabello mushroom: 2-3
- ☐ Broccoli: 1 bunch
- ☐ Sweet potatoes: 2

## Meat:

- ☐ Salmon fillets, fresh or frozen: 1+ lbs.
- ☐ Snapper fillets: 1 lb.
- ☐ Turkey, ground, organic: 1-2 lbs.
- ☐ Chicken, whole for roasting: 4-5 lbs.
- ☐ Chicken, boneless or steak for fajitas: 2 lbs.

## Dry Goods:

- ☐ Agave nectar
- ☐ Vanilla Extract
- ☐ Cinnamon
- ☐ Almond butter: 1 jar
- ☐ Coconut Milk: 1 can
- ☐ Walnuts: 1 bag
- ☐ Trail mix: 1-2 cups
- ☐ Cashews: 1 bag
- ☐ Balsamic vinegar: 1 bottle
- ☐ Olive oil: 1 bottle
- ☐ Basil: dried, 1 jar
- ☐ Onion powder: 1 jar
- ☐ Dates: Medjool, 1 package
- ☐ Sun-Dried Tomatoes: 1 package
- ☐ Garlic powder: 1 jar
- ☐ Cumin: 1 jar
- ☐ Chili powder: 1 jar
- ☐ Coconut oil: 1 jar
- ☐ Apple cider vinegar: raw, 1 bottle
- ☐ Whole grain bread: gluten free preferably
- ☐ Bars, such as LaraBars, etc..
- ☐ Popcorn: organic
- ☐ Crackers: gluten free ideally
- ☐ Salsa: fresh or in a jar
- ☐ Chickpeas: 1 can

## Dairy:

- ☐ Eggs: 1 dozen
- ☐ Yogurt: coconut milk yogurt if dairy intolerant: 3-4 cups

## Frozen goods:

- ☐ Corn, frozen: organic, 1 bag
- ☐ Peas, frozen: 1 bag

This menu plan serves 2-3 people, so adjust accordingly.

# Food Preparation Schedule

When you get home from the grocery store:

1.  Make the Creamy Basil Balsamic Vinaigrette to be used on salads for the week. You may want to double the recipe if you have a large family.

2.  Hard-boil 6-8 of the eggs to be used in salads and for breakfast. The remaining eggs will be used in the Fritatta.

3.  Preheat the oven to 350 degrees.

4.  You can go ahead and pre-cook some of the main dishes for the week. Get the whole chicken ready to be placed in the oven. See the recipe on page 144. Place the potatoes and any other vegetables you want to add in the oven to cook along with the chicken. The sweet potatoes can also be cooked at the same time.

5.  After you eat the roasted chicken for dinner, remove most of the remaining meat from the carcass and save it for salads and sand-wiches. Save the bones and make chicken broth now or freeze in a large Ziploc type bag to be made into broth another day.

6.  Lunches and breakfasts are both very easy to put together from the food that you will already have on hand.


The evening meals can be cooked each night if that works for your schedule or you can cook two times each week by cooking half of the meals each time.

## SHOPPER'S GUIDE TO PESTICIDES IN PRODUCE

### THE DIRTY DOZEN
*BUY THESE ORGANIC*

- PEACHES
- APPLES
- BELL PEPPER
- CELERY
- STRAWBERRIES
- SPINACH
- NECTARINES
- GRAPES
- POTATOES
- BLUEBERRIES
- LETTUCE
- KALE/COLLARDS

### LOWEST IN PESTICIDES
*CAN BE NON-ORGANIC*

- ONIONS
- SWEET CORN
- PINEAPPLES
- AVOCADOS
- ASPARAGUS
- PEAS
- MANGOES
- EGGPLANT
- CANTALOUPE
- KIWI
- CABBAGE
- WATERMELON
- SWEET POTATOES
- GRAPEFRUIT
- MUSHROOMS

WWW.GETPUREVITALITY.COM

# Week 2 Menu Plan

|  | **Breakfast** | **Lunch** | **Dinner** |
|---|---|---|---|
| **Mon** | Banana Nut smoothie<br><br>Snack: apple and cashews | Greek Salad with hard boiled eggs | Tarragon Chicken, steamed broccoli, and a salad |
| **Tue** | Mango Smoothie<br><br>Snack: Popcorn | Leftover chicken on mixed greens and vinaigrette | Asian Garlic Salmon, snow peas, and asparagus |
| **Wed** | Fresh fruit and a raw food bar<br><br>Snack: Trail mix and an apple | Leftover salmon on mixed greens with mung bean sprouts and a vinaigrette | Tacos With guacamole And salsa<br><br>(soak lentils) |
| **Thu** | Berry and Banana smoothie<br><br>Snack: Raw bar and some fruit | Spinach salad with hard boiled eggs, avocado, walnuts, and vegetables | Lentil Soup |
| **Fri** | Almond butter on toast and fresh fruit<br><br>Snack: apple and cashews | Leftover lentil soup and a salad | Spaghetti |
| **Sat** | Banana Nut Smoothie<br><br>Snack: berries with coconut cream | Egg salad on a bed of greens | Skip's Chicken, Zucchini and onions, and sliced tomatoes |
| **Sun** | Fritatta<br><br>Snack: apple and trail mix | (Use leftover chicken bones to make broth) Chicken salad on lettuce greens | Italian Vegetable Soup with bread and a salad |

# Shopping List for Week 2

## Produce:

- ☐ Bananas: 1 bunch
- ☐ Mango: 2
- ☐ Apples: 1 large bag
- ☐ Berries: 1 lb
- ☐ Spinach: 1 bag
- ☐ Avocados: 3-4 ripe
- ☐ Red Onion: 1
- ☐ Lettuce: 2 containers
- ☐ Yellow onion: 1 bag
- ☐ Carrots: 1 lb. bag
- ☐ Celery, 1 bag
- ☐ Yellow squash: 1 lb.
- ☐ Tomatoes: 4 large
- ☐ Garlic: 1 head
- ☐ Zucchini: 6
- ☐ Lemon: 1
- ☐ Mung bean sprouts
- ☐ Green onions: 1 bunch
- ☐ Romaine lettuce: 2-3
- ☐ Broccoli: 1 bunch
- ☐ Fresh Basil, 1 bunch
- ☐ Snow peas, 1 lb.
- ☐ Asparagus, 1 lb.

## Meat:

- ☐ Salmon fillets, fresh or frozen: 2 lbs.
- ☐ Beef or Buffalo, ground: 2 lbs.
- ☐ Turkey, ground, organic: 1-2 lbs.
- ☐ Chicken, thighs: 4 lbs.
- ☐ Chicken, whole: for broth

## Dry Goods:

- ☐ Agave nectar
- ☐ Vanilla Extract
- ☐ Cinnamon
- ☐ Almond butter: 1 jar
- ☐ Coconut Milk: 1 can
- ☐ Walnuts: 1 bag
- ☐ Trail mix: 1-2 cups
- ☐ Cashews: 1 bag
- ☐ Red wine vinegar: 1 bottle
- ☐ Olive oil: 1 bottle
- ☐ Basil: dried, 1 jar
- ☐ Onion powder: 1 jar
- ☐ Dates: Medjool, 1 package
- ☐ Lentils, 1 lb.
- ☐ Black olives
- ☐ Garlic powder: 1 jar
- ☐ Tarragon, 1 jar
- ☐ Cumin: 1 jar
- ☐ Chili powder: 1 jar
- ☐ Dijon mustard
- ☐ Coconut oil: 1 jar
- ☐ Apple cider vinegar: raw, 1 bottle
- ☐ Whole grain bread: gluten free preferably
- ☐ Bars, such as LaraBars, etc..
- ☐ Popcorn: organic
- ☐ Salsa: fresh or in a jar
- ☐ Tomatoes, canned: 3 cans
- ☐ Kidney beans, canned:1
- ☐ Garbanzo beans, canned:1

## Dairy:

- ☐ Eggs: 1 dozen
- ☐ Feta cheese, 5 oz.

## Frozen goods:

- ☐ Peas, frozen: 1 bag

# Food Preparation Schedule

1. Make a salad dressing to use for the week or just keep it simple and dress the salads with a bit of balsamic vinegar, olive oil, and sea salt.

2. The Tarragon Chicken and the Asian Garlic Salmon can be made ahead of time if necessary to save time during the week.

3. Hard boil some of the eggs for use in egg salads and the Greek salad during the week.

4. You will need to soak the lentils in water overnight on Wednesday so they are much easier to cook on Thursday.

5. Skip's Chicken is a perfect meal for the weekend as it can just slowly cook on the stove for several hours while you go about your day.

6. Save all the bones from the chicken thighs and on Sunday, you can put them in a stockpot and make chicken stock. Add more chicken to make a larger quantity.

# ~ Coconut Milk ~

Coconut milk makes a wonderful substitute for cream or milk in recipes where you want a creamy texture and rich flavor. It is a wonderful addition to both sweet and savory dishes.

- It can be used in creamy soups instead of dairy products.

- When mashing white or sweet potatoes, add coconut milk instead of regular milk or cream.

- It is wonderful in smoothies, especially ones made with tropical fruits like mango or pineapple.

- It is delicious with a little honey and vanilla stirred in and poured over fresh fruit.

- You can use it as the liquid in quick breads and muffins.

- Coconut milk ice cream is now available at many grocery stores and is a great alternative to milk-based ice creams.

# Weekly Menu Plan

|  | Breakfast | Lunch | Dinner |
|---|---|---|---|
| **Mon** |  |  |  |
| **Tue** |  |  |  |
| **Wed** |  |  |  |
| **Thu** |  |  |  |
| **Fri** |  |  |  |
| **Sat** |  |  |  |
| **Sun** |  |  |  |

Make copies of these pages to simplify meal planning and shopping.

# Shopping List

Produce:

Meat/Seafood:

Dairy/Eggs:

Frozen Foods:

Dry Goods:

Household Items:

Canned Goods:

Make copies of these pages to simplify meal planning and shopping.

# Real-Life Situations

## Eating Out

What about eating out at restaurants?  Some people may limit social events because of their new dietary rules, which can isolate them from their friends.  Your diet is not your identity.  Don't get too hung up on dogma or rules.  *Eating out is about making the best food choices you can under the circumstances.*  Your diet should not negatively impact your social life.  If it is, then you need to rethink your situation.  Life is more than food.  Make the best food choices you can and remember that *it is what you do 90% of the time that is important.*

When you go to a restaurant, you do not have to bring your own food.  That can be uncomfortable for the restaurant staff as well as the people you are dining with.  Aside from some fast food restaurants, nearly every restaurant has real food choices that you can choose from.  Try to adapt to wherever you are and do not make your friends uncomfortable.  There are usually some things you can eat.

Here are some guidelines that will enable you to enjoy eating out without worries.

Rule #1 is:  **No bread or appetizers**.  Do not eat the bread that is served as an appetizer because it is usually made with enriched flour.  Most appetizers are not healthy options.  Depending on the type of restaurant, the safest bet is to skip the appetizer and just start with a salad.  If you are starving, you can munch on some the nuts you have stashed away in your car before going in the restaurant.  This will take the edge off your hunger.

Rule #2:  **Keep it simple**.  For the main meal, keep it simple and order grilled meat or fish and 1 or 2 vegetable side dishes.  Or have an entrée salad without the cheese and croutons.  Or you could order several of the vegetable side dishes.

At a Mexican restaurant, you could order fajitas and put the meat, grilled peppers and onions on a bed of lettuce, and top it with salsa, beans, and guacamole, leaving off the tortillas and cheese. It is basically a fajita salad, and is so delicious you will not even miss the tortillas.

Rule #3: **Avoid all sauces, gravies, and soups** because they are usually loaded with MSG and can contain other problematic ingredients, such as enriched flour. Salad dressings can also be a source of unhealthy fats and MSG. Pick a vinaigrette or ask for vinegar and olive oil instead.

Rule # 4: **No fried food**. Stay away from anything breaded and fried, no matter what it is. Fried foods are very hard to digest and are loaded with harmful fats.

Rule # 5: When you are at restaurants or other social events, eat what you can and always bring a 80% chocolate bar that you can eat for dessert without feeling deprived.

## Holidays and Special Occasions

Make the best food choices you can in these situations and re-member that *it is what you do 90% of the time that is important.* Certain holidays or special occasions should be enjoyed. Eating whatever you want for Christmas and Thanksgiving is fine, and you have not fallen off the wagon. But just keep those indulgences confined to the holidays, not the entire month of December. When you give yourself permission to enjoy the holiday, it removes a lot of the guilt and shame we tend to feel for abandoning our diet temporarily. Many people give up on their strict diets during the holidays because they feel like they cannot indulge. When they do indulge, they end up throwing the baby out with the bath-water, so to speak, and abandoning their healthy diet all together.

When you are committed to eating well 90% of the time, you are free to enjoy some of your old favorites now and then. Knowing you can have something you like to eat can really make a difference in the ultimate success of your healthy diet.  The desserts in this book are so good, you will not feel deprived in the least!!

It's all about food ratios.  If you eat a lot of raw veggies with a small steak, it will digest a lot easier and you will feel a lot better than if you eat a large steak with bread or potatoes with no raw vegetables. Remember the food pyramid on page 38?  You should be eating a lot of vegetables.  They will enable your body to stay healthy.  You cannot expect vibrant health if you are eating a large piece of meat or fish and very few vegetables.

When you do indulge, rather than eating the entire chocolate bar or dessert, just have a few bites.  Or have some fruit along with it.  Take the time to savor those few bites, rather than mindlessly eating the entire thing!  Even the healthy desserts in this book can keep you from achieving vibrant health if you eat them in excess and do not eat enough vegetables.  I know those Raw Chocolate Cups are divine, but eating 8 of them a day is not a good idea.  It's all about *balance.*

Please note that if you find that your dietary indulgences are causing you to feel significantly worse or are causing intense cravings, you might need to be more careful what you eat.  That is a decision that you will have to make, depending on your current level of health.  Listen to your body and monitor how you feel, and your body will let you know.

## Food As Medicine

As you listen to your body, you will discover that certain foods may make you feel better than others.  If need to lose weight, you might find eating a higher percentage of raw foods, such as 80-90% raw, will enable the stubborn weight to fall off.  If you have IBS or digestive problems, you might find eating more soups, broths, and fermented foods are most beneficial to your body.  Those with weak digestion should not eat proteins at the same meal with starches or bread.  People with adrenal issues should not eat fruit or smoothies for breakfast, but later in the day is usually fine.  Pay attention to your body to learn what is best for you.

# Feeding Families

Changing your whole family's eating habits overnight is likely to cause loud opposition. No one likes having their favorite foods snatched away. Instead, proceed gradually and use positive motivation rather than saying how bad those foods are for you. If you tell a teenager to quit eating junk food so his schoolwork will improve, he is not likely to change. But if you guarantee more stamina for sports and less acne, you will probably get results.

- **Start fixing delicious healthy food**, like the raw chocolate pies or brownies, and let them try them without making a big deal about how healthy they are. When you make tasty alternatives, you will win them over much easier. It takes time for their tastes to change, so go very gradually and fix healthier versions of their favorites.

- **Make gradual changes**: you can mix the whole grain flour with enriched flour, rather than switching directly to whole grains. If you start with just one third of the flour as whole grain flour, and slowly increase the amount over time, usually no one will notice the change.

- **Keep healthy snacks on hand and accessible**: bowls of fruit within reach, raw nuts, dried fruit, homemade muffins, etc...

- **Visit a farm or farmer's market**. Children will probably love vegetables more if they are homegrown and fresh. Quality makes all the difference and kids can taste it.

- **Switch to raw honey, stevia or agave**. If children are resistant to eating vegetables, you can drizzle a bit of raw honey over them until they grow accustomed to them.

- **Involve your child.** Let them help you shop for healthy foods. Let them choose some items from a health food store. This gives them more control over the changes that are being made to their diet. Let them get involved in the mealtime preparations. Make it fun!

- **Add vegetables** to soups, meat dishes, and other meals. They can even be pureed and added to baked goods.

- **Try the "one bite to be polite" rule** if a child refuses to try the food you prepared. After a bite, he may decide that he likes it and will eat more or at least tolerate it without complaining. When this happens, thank him for eating it. As their taste buds change and adapt, they will find that they will start to eat these foods. But if they truly dislike the food, acknowledge their effort and do not force them to eat the food. Allow them to eat something else in the meal that you prepared. The "one bite to be polite" lesson will also teach children to show love and respect to the person who has prepared the meal.

- **Don't make another separate meal for your children**. Allow children to pick and choose what they would like to eat from what you have made. If a food is not liked by their taste buds, it may change over time. Have them try it again in a few weeks to see if they like it.

- **Avoid being too restrictive**. While we shouldn't let our children eat whatever they want all the time, we shouldn't be too restrictive either. We can control what they eat for a short time during their lives, but eventually they will be exposed to unhealthy foods. A parent's attitude about food can affect what kids will do when they grow up. If you are feeding them foods with high nutritional value most of the time, you can allow occasional treats without worry.

- **Go beyond, "Because it's good for you" comments**. It is not helpful to put "good" and "bad" labels on foods. Get specific when you talk about what the foods do for your health, for example, "white bread zaps energy from our bodies", "sugar can cause cavities and damage our teeth", "fish makes us smart", "spinach makes us strong" or "this food makes us healthy and strong but this food makes us get sick".

- **Start a garden**. As children learn how plants grow, they will be more inclined to eat the food they so carefully tended.

- **Get greens into children by making green smoothies**. Blend some of their favorite fruits with a handful of spinach, put it onto an opaque cup and serve with a straw. If you add blackberries or blueberries to it, it will turn purple and they won't be able to tell the greens are in it. You can also make them into popsicles. When I make a morning green smoothie for me or my husband, I will take the rest and put it into popsicle molds for my daughter's after school snack. It is an easy, healthy snack and she loves it!

- **Make food fun!** Get creative. One parent told me that she would put various cut up vegetables on a plate and let her children get creative and make shapes or animals with them, with understanding that they would have to eat what they made. What a great idea!

- **Don't make it a battle**. Remember, food is what gives us our nourishment. The most healthy meal eaten with hostility is counterproductive to health. Meals are meant to be shared with love and fellowship with those we care about. Do not let food bring division into your family. Those relationships are just as important to your health and wellbeing as the food you prepare.

- **Your support is crucial**. You cannot expect your children to change their eating habits without also eating well yourself. As a parent, you are the one who needs to set the example.

- **Have a game plan**. Your child will be offered candy and sweets at nearly every turn in our society. You need to be prepared for this. In our home, we let our child trade in the candy she gets for a toy or something else. We ask the church or school teachers to give her stickers or toys instead of candy. While we do let her have candy occasionally, we have found that when it is eaten more once or twice a month, it causes intense sugar cravings. Sugar can be addictive. So, try to keep it to a minimum.

# Healthy Lunchbox Ideas for Children

To make sure your children get a well-balanced diet, have a main entrée item, a side item, and a snack. Pick one item from the first group and 2 from the second group to pack for lunch.

## Main Dish

A sandwich or wrap made with 100% whole grain bread can include these fillings:

- Almond butter (or other nut butter) and raw honey or banana
- Nitrate-free natural deli meat and lettuce, avocado, tomato, etc..
- Grilled cheese
- Chicken Salad
- Egg salad
- Raw cheese and natural pepperoni
- Refried beans and raw cheese
- Hummus and lettuce or spinach

Another option is leftovers or soup in a thermos.

## Side Items/Snacks

- Applesauce
- Fresh fruit or fruit leathers
- Gluten-free or whole grain cookies or bars, such as Larabars
- Trail mix or granola
- Dates Candy (page 179)
- Raw vegetables cut up with a dip or hummus
- Vegetable or bean salad
- Gluten-free or whole grain crackers and raw cheese
- Yogurt (dairy, or non-dairy yogurt)
- Beef jerky
- Gluten-free or whole grain brownies, muffins, banana bread, etc...

# Tracking Your Progress

As you change your diet, it is helpful to keep track of all the benefits you are experiencing.  Fill out this form a few months after completing most of the Baby Steps.  Compare this to the first health inventory form you filled out and you will realize how far you have come.

What changes have you noticed over the past few months of eating well?

_____

_____

_____

Current weight:_____ Blood pressure:_____ Blood sugar:_____

Current symptoms:  (check all that apply and explain)
- ☐ Energy: 1 (low) - 5 (high):_____
- ☐ Sleep (how many hours and quality):_____
- ☐ Mental /Mood:_____
- ☐ Skin:_____
- ☐ Digestion:_____
- ☐ Elimination (how often are your bowel movements?):_____
- ☐ Pain level:_____
- ☐ Allergies (food or environmental):_____
- ☐ Male/Female organs:_____
- ☐ Respiratory system:_____
- ☐ Immune system:_____
- ☐ Stress level:_____

Physical activity (type and how often):_____

## Food Intake

Breakfast:_____ Time:_____

Lunch:_____ Time:_____

Snack:_____ Time:_____

Dinner:_____ Time:_____

Water intake:_____

Other beverages:_____

_____

# Supplements

Most people benefit from adding some supplements to their diet. Although it is certainly ideal to get all of our nutrition from food, it is becoming increasingly difficult due to low soil fertility, shipping produce long distances, and over-processing.

Here are some basics that you may want to consider:

- **A Multi-vitamin**: Look for one that is food-based and contains vitamins, minerals, trace minerals, and antioxidants.

- **Probiotics:** Probiotics provide beneficial bacteria that aid in digestion, strengthen the immune system, and support overall health. Make sure they have been kept refrigerated for maximum potency.

- **Digestive Enzymes**: A good quality digestive enzyme supplement is important to take when you eat meals of mostly cooked foods. It will help you digest the food more efficiently and helps reduce indigestion, bloating, and other digestive complaints.

- **Cod Liver Oil**: Cod liver oil is rich in Vitamins A and D, which are important for the absorption of minerals, resistance to sickness, and the health of the bones.

For more details on supplements for your particular health condition, please see an alternative healthcare practitioner.

# Beverages
# &
# Smoothies

# Smoothies & Shakes

## Banana Nut Smoothie
1 large banana
2 Tbsp. almond or peanut butter
1/2 tsp. vanilla extract
2 Medjool dates or dried fruit or agave to sweeten
1/8 tsp. cinnamon
1-2 cups almond milk or filtered water
Handful of spinach (optional for a green smoothie)

Blend and serve immediately.   Makes 1 serving.

## Mango Smoothie
1 ripe mango
1/2 cup  raspberries or 1/2 cup cherries
1/3 cup coconut milk or 2 Tbsp. coconut butter
3 Tbsp. nut butter
1 tsp. vanilla extract
Honey or agave to taste
1 cup almond milk or filtered water

Blend and serve.  Makes 1 serving.

## Pear Maple Green Smoothie
1 ripe pear
3 dried figs, chopped
3 Tbsp. nut butter
1/2 tsp. vanilla extract
1/4 tsp. cinnamon
1/2 tsp. maple extract (or use maple syrup to sweeten)
Handful of spinach
1 cup almond milk or coconut milk

Blend  in a high speed blender and serve. Makes 1 serving.

## Banana Berry Shake

1 large banana
2 Tbsp. almond or raw cashew butter
1 cup almond milk
1/2 tsp. vanilla extract
3-4 large strawberries

Blend and serve immediately.   Makes 1 serving.

## Energizing Green Smoothie

1 frozen banana (or 1 cup of any frozen fruit)
1 large kale leaf (or a handful of any leafy green vegetable)
1 tsp. vanilla extract
2 dates or dried figs (optional)
1 cup almond milk
Stevia to taste

Blend in a high speed blender.   Add water to thin if necessary.
Serve immediately.   Makes 1 serving.

## Shakeology

Want to boost the nutrient density of your smoothies?  Shakeology is a shake mix that contains over 70 ingredients!  It has vitamins, minerals, superfoods, herbs, probiotics, digestive enzymes, protein, and fiber. All you do is blend it with some almond milk and fruit.

It is great for a quick meal on the go or for people looking to boost their nutrient intake.  It helps reduce cholesterol levels, increase energy, and help control cravings.  For more information, see www.getpurevitality.com

# Juicing Recipes

| | |
|---|---|
| 1 celery stalk<br>1/2 beet<br>1 large carrot<br>1/2 apple | 3 large carrots<br>1 large cucumber<br>2~3 kale leaves<br>1/2 lemon |
| 1/2 cucumber<br>1 large handful of spinach<br>1 large carrot<br>1/2 apple | 8 kale leaves<br>1/2 bunch parsley<br>3 stalks celery<br>1 apple<br>1 lemon |
| 4 carrots<br>1 large cucumber<br>  or zucchini<br>1 apple<br>1 lemon | 3 large carrots<br>1/2 cucumber<br>1/2 celery stalk<br>1 handful of spinach |
| 5 carrots<br>1/2 fennel bulb | 3 carrots<br>1 zucchini<br>1 apple |
| 6 carrots<br>1/2 beet<br>1 zucchini<br>1/2 lime | 6 carrots<br>1/2 lemon<br>1 zucchini<br>A handful of spinach<br>1 inch of gingerroot<br>1/2 apple |

**Each recipe makes about 1 large serving**

# 30-Second Nut Milk

2-3 heaping Tbsp. of raw nut butter
1 Tbsp. coconut butter (or 1/4 cup coconut milk)
1/2 tsp. vanilla extract
Pinch of salt
Sweetener to taste (2 Tbsp. agave or 3-4 drops stevia extract)
1 1/2-2 cups filtered water

Put all ingredients into a blender and blend well.

# Almond Milk

1 cup raw almonds, soaked in water for 4 hours or more
3-4 cups filtered water
Agave or stevia to taste
A pinch of sea salt
1/2 tsp. vanilla extract

Drain water from almonds.  In a blender, blend the nuts with the water and remaining ingredients on high for about 2 minutes.

# Maple Pecan Milk

1 cup raw pecans, soaked in water for 2 hours or more, and drained
3 1/2 cups filtered water
Agave or stevia to taste
2 Tbsp. coconut butter
2 tsp. vanilla extract
1 tsp. maple extract
1/2 tsp. cinnamon
Pinch of sea salt

Blend all ingredients until smooth.  Strain if desired.

# Brazil Nut Milk

1 cup brazil nuts, soaked in water a few hours, then drained
3 cups filtered water
Sweetener to taste
Pinch of sea salt
1 tsp. vanilla extract
Pinch of cinnamon

Place all ingredients into a blender  and blend until smooth.

# Beverages

## Lemonade

5 lemons, juiced
5 limes, juiced
5 oranges, juiced
3 quarts filtered water
Honey or agave to taste

Combine all ingredients in a
gallon container and mix well.

## Banana Egg Nog

2 farm fresh organic eggs
2 small bananas
1 1/2 cups of almond or coconut mi
1/2 tsp. vanilla
A pinch of freshly grated nutmeg

Puree in blender and serve
immediately.   Serves 1-2

## Mango Lasse

1 cup plain yogurt
1 ripe mango, peeled and cut up
1 tsp. vanilla extract
1/2 tsp. cinnamon
1 cup orange juice

Blend until smooth and serve.
Serves 1-2

## Apple Spice Lemonade

3 apples
1 whole lemon
1 inch piece of gingerroot

Juice all ingredients and enjoy!

## Peppermint Tea

1 heaping tsp. licorice root
2 heaping tsp. peppermint leaves
2 cups filtered water

Place herbs in a saucepan and
add water.  Bring just to a boil,
cover, and remove from heat.  Let
sit for 5 minutes and strain.

## Chocolate Milk

2 cups nut milk (see previous pg.)
2 Tbsp. cocoa powder or carob
1 tsp. vanilla extract
Pinch of cinnamon
Pinch of salt
Stevia or agave to taste

Blend all ingredients in a blender.

## Ginger Lemonade

8 carrots
2 lemons
1x2 inch piece of ginger root
Stevia or agave to taste
1 cup pineapple juice (optional)

Juice the carrots, lemons, and
ginger.  This should make about 2
cups of concentrated juice.  Add 6
cups of filtered water to make
1/2 gallon and sweeten to taste.

## Holiday Egg Nog

I cup of almond or coconut milk
1 egg yolk
1 date
6 drops stevia extract
1/2 tsp. vanilla
A pinch of freshly grated nutmeg

Puree in blender and serve
immediately.   Serves 1-2

# Appetizers
# &
# Snacks

# Crispy Nuts

Nuts that are raw, not roasted, are more nutritious and have their live enzymes still intact, which facilitates their digestion. Roasted nuts that have been heated at high temperatures are hard to digest, lack the beneficial enzymes, and can contain rancid, unhealthy fats. Crispy nut recipes use raw nuts that have been soaked in water and then dehydrated to make them crisp. This process preserves the enzymes and nutrients in the raw nut and makes it more digestible.

---

## Crispy Nuts Basic Recipe (adapted from Nourishing Traditions)

4 cups nuts (almonds, pecans, hazelnuts, pumpkin seeds, walnuts, etc)

1 Tbsp. sea salt

Place nuts and salt in a large bowl. Fill with filtered water to cover the nuts and stir to dissolve the salt. Let stand at room temperature for at least 6-7 hours. Drain in a colander and spread out on a mesh dehydrator tray. Dehydrate at 100 degrees for 24-48 hours (depending on the humidity in your area), or until totally dry and crispy. Store in airtight containers in the pantry, except for walnuts, which must be refrigerated.

Makes 4 cups

---

## Variations:

**Spicy Nuts:** After draining the nuts or seeds from the water, place in dehydrator and dry them for a couple of hours. Mix 2 Tbsp. minced chives, 2 Tbsp. paprika, 1 Tbsp. garlic powder, 1/2 Tbsp. onion powder, 1 tsp sea salt, a pinch of cayenne powder, and 2 Tbsp. olive oil in a large bowl. Add the partially dried nuts/seeds and stir to coat. Place them back in the dehydrator and continue to dry until crispy.

**Seasoned Nuts**: After placing the nuts in the dehydrator for a couple hours, remove and coat with 2 Tbsp. garlic powder, 4 Tbsp. onion powder, 2 Tbsp. olive oil, and enough soy sauce to make a thick paste. Return to dehydrator until crispy.

## Power Bars

2 1/2 cups  raw almonds

1/2 cup flax meal

1/2 cup shredded coconut

1/2 tsp. sea salt

1/2 cup coconut oil, melted

5 drops stevia extract

1 Tbsp. agave or honey

1 Tbsp. vanilla extract

3/4 cup dried fruit (raisins, figs, etc..) chopped

1/2 dark chocolate bar (optional for topping)

Combine first 5 ingredients in a food processor and pulse to mix for about 30 seconds.  Combine the coconut oil, stevia, agave, and vanilla in a bowl and add to food processor mixture.  Add the dried fruit and pulse the mixture until it starts to become a coarse paste.  Press into a 8 x 8 baking dish and chill in the refrigerator for 1 hour.  Top with melted chocolate bar and cut into bars.  Store in the refrigerator.

## Coconut Fudge Balls

1 cup dried coconut, finely shredded

3 soft dates

2 Tbsp. cocoa or carob powder

1 Tbsp. cinnamon

1/2 tsp. vanilla extract

1 Tbsp. coconut oil

Pinch of sea salt

2 Tbsp. dried coconut, finely shredded, for topping

Combine all ingredients, except for the last ingredient, in a food processor and process until it holds together.  Shape into 1 1/2 inch balls and roll in coconut.

# Truffles

1 cup almonds, ground fine in food processor

1/2 cup  raisins or dried apricots or figs

1/2 tsp. cinnamon

1 tsp. vanilla

1 tsp. maple extract, optional

A pinch of salt

Grind all ingredients together in a food processor until it starts to clump together and form a ball.  If it does not clump together, add a couple tsp of water until it does.  Form into balls (or press into a pan and chill, then cut into bars).  Store in refrigerator.

---

# High-Energy Truffles

2 cups raw almonds or other nuts, ground in food processor

1/2 cup golden raisins or other dried fruit

2 large golden dried figs or other dried fruit

1/2 cup Siberian Ginseng root powder

1/8 cup bee pollen

2 Tbsp. vanilla extract

1 tsp. cinnamon

4 Tbsp. coconut butter

1 Tbsp. flax oil

1/4 tsp. sea salt

1-2 Tbsp. water (optional)

Place all ingredients in a food processor and process until the mixture starts to hold together.  Add the optional water if needed.  Form into balls and store in the refrigerator.

Note: Bee pollen may cause allergic reactions in sensitive individuals.

## Sesame Truffles

*Sesame seeds are a rich source of calcium and other minerals. These truffles are a great way to increase your calcium intake.*

1/2 cup sesame seeds,

4 dried figs

1 tsp. vanilla extract

Pinch salt

Pinch of cinnamon

Grind up the sesame seeds in a coffee grinder.  Place all ingredients together in a food processor and process for a minute or until it can old it's shape when formed into a ball.  Form into balls (or press into a pan and chill, then cut into bars).  Store in refrigerator.

## Cinnamon Apple Chips

3 or more apples, peeled, cored, and sliced (Pink Lady is our favorite)

1 Tbsp. cinnamon

1/2 Tbsp. unrefined sugar, such as Rapadura brand

1/4 tsp. allspice

An apple/peeler/corer/slicer tool available from cooking stores makes preparation a breeze.

Mix the spices and sugar together on a plate.  Roll the outside edge of the apple slices in the spices and lay slices on mesh dehydrator sheets.  Dehydrate at 100-110 degrees until dry and crisp, 12-24 hours.  Store in an airtight container in the pantry.

# Nacho Kale Chips

Nacho Sauce recipe from page 126, double the recipe if the kale is
     large

1 bunch of kale


Wash kale and tear off stem into bite sized pieces and place in
a large bowl.  Pour the Nacho Sauce over it and stir to coat each piece.
It should be heavily coated.

Place onto mesh dehydrator screen trays and dehydrate at

100-110 degrees for 6-12 hours, or until completely dry and crispy.

Store in an airtight container in the pantry.  Makes about 1
gallon.

---

# Grain-free Granola

1 apple, chopped

1 cup dried fruit, such as dates, figs, apricots, raisins, etc..

1/2 cup honey or other sweetener

2 Tbsp. lemon juice

1 Tbsp. vanilla extract

2 tsp. cinnamon

2 tsp. sea salt

7 cups raw nuts and seeds, soaked in water a few hours, drained

1 cup dried cranberries

In a food processor, place the apple, dried fruit, sweetener,
lemon juice, vanilla, cinnamon, salt, and a 1/4 cup of the nuts/seeds
and grind until completely smooth.  Transfer to a bowl.  Drain the nuts
and seeds and place in food processor to coarsely chop.  Add to the
bowl with the apple mixture, add the cranberries and stir well.  Spread
on dehydrator trays and dry until crisp.

# Baba Ghanouj ~ (Roasted Eggplant Dip)

2 medium eggplants

2-3 Tbsp. olive oil

6-7 large cloves garlic, sliced

1 medium onion, chopped and sautéed until carmelized

1/2 tsp. cumin

1/2 cup tahini

Juice of 1 lemon

Sea salt to taste

Pinch of smoked paprika

### Optional ingredients:

4 green onions, chopped

1/2 bunch cilantro, chopped

1 green jalepeno pepper, seeded and minced

1 red bell pepper, diced

Cut the eggplants in half lengthwise, score the flesh all the way to the skin in a 1 inch grid. Drizzle with olive oil and push sliced garlic into the cuts and roast at 375 degrees for about 1 hour or until it is browned.

Scrape the inside flesh out of the eggplants when cool enough to handle. Discard the skins. Add the sautéed onion, cumin, tahini, lemon juice, paprika, and salt and mix well.

Use this recipe as a dip for bread or raw vegetables.

Optional ingredients can be stirred in until well combined and served at room temperature.

## Rosemary Crackers

2 cups walnuts, soaked in water for a few hours

1/2 cup sunflower seeds, soaked in water a few hours

1 clove garlic, minced

3 green onions, chopped

1 Tbsp. fresh rosemary, minced

2 tsp. red wine vinegar

1 Tbsp. honey

1 tsp. sea salt

1/2 cup whole flaxseeds, ground finely in a coffee grinder

Drain the nuts and seeds in a colander. Place in a food processor along with the rest of the ingredients, except for the flaxseeds. Process to form a coarse paste. Stir or pulse in the flaxmeal. Spread the mixture onto non-stick dehydrator sheets about 1/4 inch thick with a rubber spatula. Score into rectangles with a knife. Dehydrate at around 100 degrees for about 12-24 hours, turning over once halfway through the drying time. Dry until crisp.

Makes about 20 crackers.

# Salsa

4 large tomatoes, diced

1/2 large sweet onion, minced

3 cloves garlic, minced

2/3 cup chopped cilantro, optional

1 jalapeno pepper, seeded and minced

2 Tbsp. lime juice

Sea salt to taste

Combine all ingredients in a bowl, adding jalapeno 2 teaspoons at a time, tasting to determine how hot you like it.. Store in the refrigerator.

# Guacamole

3 ripe avocados

1 Tbsp. lime juice

Sea salt to taste

Cut avocados in half and remove the seed. Scoop out the flesh and place in a bowl. Add lime juice and mash the avocado with a fork. Stir in sea salt to taste.

# Mexican Layered Dip

28 oz. can of refried beans or 4 cups cooked beans, mashed

4 avocados, mashed with 2 tsp. lemon juice and 1/2 tsp. salt added

8 oz sour cream or plain yogurt with 2 tsp. chili powder and 1 tsp. garlic salt mixed in or skip the dairy and use Salsa for this layer

8 oz. shredded cheese

1 bunch green onions, chopped

2 tomatoes, chopped

Chopped cilantro

On a large platter, spread the beans in an even layer, top with avocado mixture, then the sour cream mixture. Sprinkle on the cheese, green onions, tomatoes, and cilantro. Serve with tortilla chips.

# Hummus

*Hummus makes a great dip for vegetables or flatbread or as a sandwich spread, or instead of the marinara sauce on a vegetable pizza.*

2 cups cooked chickpeas, drained

1/8 cup tahini, or ground sesame seeds

2 cloves garlic, minced

1 Tbsp. lemon juice

1/2 cup water

1 tsp. cumin

2 tsp. sea salt or Herbamare

1 Tbsp. freshly minced parsley, optional

1/4 cup olive oil

1/2 tsp. hot sauce, optional

Place the chickpeas, tahini, garlic, lemon juice, water, cumin, salt, parsley, olive oil, and hot sauce in a food processor and process until the mixture is well blended but slightly coarse.    Makes 3 cups

---

# Popcorn

For the stovetop, heat a pan with a lid on medium-high heat. Add 2 Tbsp. of coconut oil and 1/2 cup popcorn to the pan. Put on the lid and hold the handle and lid of the pan (with hot pads if necessary) and start shaking back and forth over the burner until the popcorn pops and then starts to slow down it's popping. Remove from heat and add sea salt to taste. For electric air poppers, follow manufacturer's instructions to pop. Add melted coconut oil and sea salt to taste.

## Variation:  Pizza Popcorn

Mix the following ingredients into a large bowl of fresh popcorn:

4 Tbsp. melted coconut oil

2 Tbsp. nutritional yeast (found in a health food store)

1 tsp. onion powder

1 tsp. sea salt, or to taste

2 tsp. Pizza Seasoning herbs by Frontier Herbs

## Popcorn Variation: Spicy Chili Popcorn

Mix the freshly popped popcorn with 3-4 Tbsp. of coconut oil. Mix the following ingredients into a small bowl, then mix into popcorn:

2 Tbsp. nutritional yeast (found in a health food store)

2 tsp. paprika

2 tsp. chili powder

1/2 tsp. garlic powder

Cayenne pepper to taste

1-2 tsp. sea salt, or to taste

# Quick, High-Energy Snack Ideas

- Raw apples with nut butter
- Fresh fruit and raw nuts or cheese
- Tortilla chips and salsa
- Trail mix
- Popcorn made with coconut oil and sea salt
- Smoothie ingredients made into popsicles
- Homemade jerky
- Power bars (see recipe pg.89 ) and fruit
- Carrot sticks or red bell peppers and hummus
- Whole grain crackers and raw cheese
- Plain yogurt sweetened with honey, stevia, or agave and fresh fruit

# Breakfasts
# &
# Brunch

# Quick and Easy Breakfast Ideas

No time to sit and eat? No problem.  Here are some easy to make breakfast ideas.  Skipping breakfast is not a good idea (see below).

- Smoothies (see recipes on page 82 )

- Fresh fruit chopped and put in a bowl, topped with nuts

- Nut butter on whole grain bread, sliced banana on top, drizzled with honey

- Hard boiled eggs, a piece of fruit, and a handful of crackers

- Raw cheese, grapes, and a piece of whole grain bread toasted

- Whole grain frozen waffle, toasted, and spread with nut butter and applesauce

- Whole grain pita bread stuffed with cottage cheese and sliced peaches or berries and drizzled with honey

- Granola bar or raw food bar topped with nut butter

- Yogurt with agave stirred in and topped with fresh fruit

- Spinach salad topped with sliced red onion, chopped avocado, and leftover grilled chicken or other meat and a vinaigrette

- Whole grain tortilla, sprinkled with raw cheddar cheese and green apple slices,  or banana slices and nut butter, rolled up

Skipping breakfast can have a major impact on the rest of your day.  Here's why:  Blood sugar (glucose) is the fuel for every single cell in your body.  So of course you want your fuel supply to be constant all day long.  Eating meals at regular intervals throughout the day is necessary to maintain your energy levels.

Typical breakfast foods - cold cereal, bagels, donuts, pancakes, waffles, etc...- are all high in sugars and simple carbohydrates which cause the blood sugar to spike up then crash.  When your blood sugar drops too low, many symptoms can occur.  The first symptoms to set in are usually mental difficulties, because the brain requires a lot of fuel to do it's job.  The brain also requires amino acids which come from protein, not carbohydrates.  You may have trouble concentrating, being forgetful, or feeling mentally dull.  Try one of these delicious recipes for breakfast instead!

# Buckwheat Cereal

8 cups raw buckwheat (the kind that can sprout)

1 cup slivered almonds

1/2 cup other nuts (optional)

3/4 cup raisins or other dried fruit

1 cup coconut oil, melted

1/2 cup honey or other sweetener

1 tsp. vanilla

Pinch of cinnamon

Pinch of sea salt

Soak the buckwheat in water to cover for 3-5 hours, then pour into a colander to drain. Set over a large bowl and rinse the buckwheat a couple times a day until it starts to sprout. When the buckwheat has sprouts that are about 1/8- 1/4 inch long, place it in a dehydrator (set at 100 degrees) or an oven set at 150 degrees and let dry until crunchy. Store in an airtight container in pantry.

To use as a cereal, the dehydrated buckwheat is tossed with a sauce and served like a cereal or granola.

To make the sauce, combine the coconut oil, honey, vanilla, cinnamon, and salt and pour over the buckwheat, stirring well to coat. Add nuts and dried fruit. Serve with almond milk or top with fresh chopped fruit and eat like granola.

Makes 8 cups.

Note: This keeps well in an airtight container in the pantry for a few days, but it tastes best when the buckwheat and the sauce are stored separately and mix together just before serving.

# Cereal

1/2 cup nuts

4 Tbsp. shredded coconut

2 Tbsp. sesame seeds

1/2 cup dried fruit

1/4 tsp. cinnamon

Pinch of salt

Put all ingredients in a food processor and grind until coarsely ground. Put in a bowl and top with chopped fresh fruit and serve with almond milk.

Serves 1-2

---

# Fruit Parfait

2 Tbsp. flax seeds

1/4 tsp. cinnamon

1 cup fresh fruit

1/3 cup coconut cream

1/2 tsp. vanilla extract

1/4 cup nuts

Grind the flax seeds in a coffee grinder until it resembles a fine meal. Stir in cinnamon and put in a bowl. Place fruit on top of the flax meal. Mix the vanilla into the coconut cream and sweeten if desired. Pour this over the fruit and flax meal and top with the nuts. Serve immediately.

Serves 1

# Almond Flour Pancakes

2 cups almond flour (process as fine as possible in food processor or
        coffee grinder and sift to remove larger pieces), or half almond
        flour and half rice flour

1 cup coconut milk, almond milk, or water

1 tsp. baking powder

½ tsp. salt

½ cup applesauce or 1 Tbsp. honey

2 beaten eggs

1/2+ cup frozen blueberries

1 tsp. vanilla extract

Combine all ingredients and stir well. Fold in blueberries. Cook on a griddle or frying pan in coconut oil.   Serves 2

---

# Quinoa Breakfast Porridge

*Soak the quinoa overnight for a hearty and healthy breakfast the next day!*

2 cups quinoa, soaked in water to cover overnight

2 cups almond milk

1/4-1/2 tsp. cinnamon

1/2 cup raisins or chopped dried figs

Pinch of salt

Honey, agave, or stevia to taste

Rinse and drain quinoa in a fine-mesh strainer until the water runs clear. Put into a saucepan and add the almond milk, cinnamon, raisins, and salt. Bring to a boil, then reduce heat and simmer for 20 minutes.

Serve with extra sweetener if desired and any other toppings such as coconut cream, butter, nuts, etc..

Serves 2-3

# Waffles

3/4 cup rice flour

1 tsp. baking powder

Pinch of sea salt

1 tsp. unrefined sugar, such as Rapadura, or agave

1 egg, separated

1 Tbsp. coconut oil

3/4 cup coconut milk

Mix the flour with the baking powder, sea salt and sugar if using. Mix the egg yolk with the melted coconut oil, milk, and agave (if not using Rapadura). Combine the dry ingredients with the wet ingredients. Beat the egg white until stiff and fold into the batter.

Cook on a preheated waffle iron and serve immediately. Or let cool on wire racks and store in freezer for future meals.

## Variation: Gingerbread Waffles

Substitute 1/4 cup of blackstrap molasses for the unrefined sugar. And stir 1 tsp. cinnamon and 1/2 tsp. ginger into the dry ingredients.

# Oatmeal

2 cups gluten-free rolled oats or steel cut oats

Filtered water

1 tsp. sea salt

Ideally, the night before, place the oats in a bowl and cover with filtered water. Cover, and let stand at room temperature overnight. Cook or refrigerate until ready to use. To cook, add 1 cup of soaked oatmeal to 1/2-3/4 cup water or milk (depending on the consistency), bring to a boil, reduce heat, and simmer several minutes. Remove from heat and let stand for a few minutes. Serve with butter or coconut cream and a natural sweetener like honey, maple syrup, or agave.

Optional ingredients to stir in: raisins, applesauce with cinnamon, natural fruit preserves and nuts, ground flax seeds, or fresh fruit.

---

# Muffins

2 ½ c almond flour ( or half rice flour)

¼ c sunflower oil, coconut oil, or butter

4 Tbsp agave nectar or honey

½ tsp baking soda

¼ tsp. sea salt

3 eggs

½ c+ raisins (or blueberries)

2 tsp. vanilla extract

2 tsp. almond extract (omit if using blueberries)

1 Tbsp. cinnamon

Grind enough almonds in food processor to equal 2 ½ cups. Add baking soda, sea salt and cinnamon to taste. Add raisins to this mix as well and stir a bit to combine ingredients. In a separate bowl, combine eggs, agave nectar, sunflower oil, vanilla and almond extract. Mix liquid ingredients with a whisk until well blended and pour into dry ingredients. Stir until well mixed. Spoon into paper lined muffin tins. (Makes 12 regular sized or 24 mini sized.) Bake in preheated 350 degree oven for 15-20 minutes. They will puff up and I check for doneness by poking with a metal kebob skewer. If it comes out clean, they are done.

## Pancakes

2 cups whole grain gluten-free flour

2 tsp. baking powder

1/4 tsp. sea salt

1 Tbsp. honey or agave

2 eggs

1 1/2 to 2 cups almond milk or coconut milk

2 Tbsp. melted butter or coconut oil

Heat a griddle or large skillet over medium  low heat while you make the batter.  Mix the dry ingredients together.  Beat the eggs into 1 1/2 cups of milk, then stir in the oil.  Add the wet ingredients to the dry ingredients.  If it is too thick, add more milk.

Place a teaspoon of oil or butter in the pan and then add a ladle of batter, making the pancakes any size you like.  Flip them when bubbles appear on the surface of the pancake.  Cook on the second side a few minutes or until lightly browned.

Makes 4-6 servings.

## Other pancake additions:

- Stir in 1 cup frozen blueberries into the batter

- Add 1 1/2 cups mashed or pureed fruit, and reduce the flour by 1/2 cup and add another egg.

## Turkey Breakfast Sausage

1 lb. ground turkey

1 small onion, finely chopped or 1 tsp. onion powder

1/4 tsp. each cumin, marjoram, pepper, and ginger

1/2 tsp. each dried basil, thyme, and sage

2 tsp. sea salt or Herbamare

2 Tbsp. ground flax seeds

1 egg, lightly beaten

2 Tbsp. butter or oil

Mix all ingredients, except butter, and form into patties. Melt butter in pan over medium heat and cook patties in butter for several minutes per side or until done. These can be frozen , wrapped separately, in an airtight container. Serves 3-4

## Frittata

*All sorts of vegetables can be used in a frittata– use whatever you have.*

3 Tbsp. olive oil

1 onion or leek, chopped

1 Tbsp. minced garlic, optional

2 Tbsp. fresh parsley, chopped (or other herbs)

1/2 cups chopped cooked vegetables or spinach (optional)

Salt and pepper

4 eggs

Heat an oven-proof skillet over medium heat and add 2 Tbsp. olive oil. Sauté the onion until it softens and then add the garlic and parsley or herbs and turn heat down to medium-low.

If using cooked vegetables or leafy greens, add the vegetables and turn the heat down to low after the vegetables are warmed. Beat the eggs with almond milk, salt and pepper. Pour eggs into the skillet and use a spoon to distribute the vegetables evenly. Cook until the eggs are barely set, 5 to 10 minutes. Place under the broiler for a minute to set the eggs on the top if needed. Grate cheese over the top and serve warm or at room temperature.    Serves 2

# Notes

# Salads,
# Dressings
# &
# Sauces

# ~ How to Build a Great Salad ~

In order to enjoy eating more raw vegetables, you need to be able to make a great tasting salad. A great salad can be made from any number of ingredients, but they need to be fresh for the best flavor. Great salads have a variety of ingredients that add depth to their flavor. More than just iceburg lettuce and tomatoes....salads offer the ultimate in creativity. You can mix any number of fresh vegetables and other ingredients for a simply stunning salad combination. For example:

- **Vegetables:** Greens (romaine, spring mix, spinach, etc...), cucumber, peas, red bell pepper, tomatoes, avocado, red onion, jicama, sun-dried tomatoes, corn, beans, broccoli, cauliflower, carrots, celery, olives, sprouts, etc...

- **Something with crunch:** croutons, nuts, tortilla chips, etc..

- **Something sweet:** sliced strawberries, raisins, citrus sections, pineapple, apple, grapes, etc...

- **Some protein:** crumbled cheeses, leftover grilled chicken or steak cut into bite sized pieces, salad shrimp, garbanzo beans, lentils, black beans, hard boiled eggs, nuts, seeds, etc....

For a Mexican inspired salad, use spring mix lettuces with chopped red bell pepper, tomatoes, avocados, green onions, jicama, cilantro, black beans or chicken, crumbled tortilla chips, and a great dressing such as the Honey-Lime Vinaigrette or just salsa and guacamole as the dressing.

Another combination is spring mix with shredded carrots, chopped avocado, thinly sliced red onion, some sunflower sprouts, a handful of pecans, some raisins, and the Basil Vinaigrette.

You don't even need lettuce for a tasty salad. Just cut up various vegetables: zucchini, broccoli or cauliflower, tomato, carrot, and red onion and marinate in an Italian Dressing for a few hours.

For an Asian inspired salad, use a combination of shredded napa cabbage with other vegetables such as chopped green onion, grated daikon radish, snow peas, grated carrot, mushrooms, mung bean sprouts, and top with broiled salmon and the Asian Ginger Dressing.

# Dressings

## Basil Vinaigrette

3/4 cup extra virgin olive oil

1/4 cup balsamic vinegar

1/2 tsp. dried basil

1/4 tsp. garlic powder

1/4 tsp. onion powder

1 Tbsp. Dijon mustard

1 tsp. fresh lemon juice

1/2 tsp. honey or 2 drops stevia extract

1/4 tsp. sea salt or Herbamare

1/8 tsp. freshly ground pepper

Combine all ingredients in a glass jar with a tight fitting lid and shake to combine or use a whisk. Store at room temperature and shake before using. Makes 1 cup.

## Italian Dressing

1 1/3 cups cold pressed olive oil

1/2 cup raw apple cider vinegar or raw red wine vinegar

1/4 cup grated Parmesan cheese

1 Tbsp. raw honey or agave

2 tsp. sea salt or Herbamare

1 tsp. celery salt

1/2 tsp. pepper

1/2 tsp. dry mustard

1 clove garlic, minced

Combine all ingredients in a glass jar with a tight fitting lid and shake to combine or use a whisk. Store at room temperature and shake before using. Makes 1 3/4 cup.

## Asian Ginger Dressing

3 cloves garlic, minced

2 Tbsp. fresh ginger root, minced

3/4 cup olive oil

1/4 cup raw apple cider vinegar

1/2 cup soy sauce

3 Tbsp. raw honey or agave

1/3 cup filtered water

Combine all ingredients in a glass jar with a tight fitting lid and shake to combine or use a whisk.  Store at room temperature and shake before using.

This dressing goes nicely on a salad of thinly sliced napa cabbage topped with grated carrot, diakon radish, bell pepper, red onion, etc...

---

## Honey Lime Vinaigrette

1 clove garlic, minced

3 Tbsp. fresh lime juice

3 Tbsp. fresh orange juice

1 tsp. onion powder

1 Tbsp. honey

1/2 tsp. ground cumin

1/4 cup olive oil

Salt to taste

Combine all ingredients in a glass jar with a tight fitting lid and shake to combine or use a whisk.  Store at room temperature and shake before using.

# Mayonnaise

2 egg yolks, at room temperature

1 tsp. Dijon mustard

1 Tbsp. fresh lemon juice or wine vinegar

1 cup mild oil, such as avocado or sunflower

1/2 tsp. sea salt

In a blender or food processor, place the egg yolks, mustard, lemon juice, and salt. Turn on the motor on low and immediately begin to add the oil in a thin and steady stream. When all of the oil has been added, quickly turn off the machine. The mixture should be thick with all of the oil blended in. Taste and add more salt if necessary.

# Creamy Parmesan Dressing

1/2 cup mayonnaise

1/4 cup grated Parmesan cheese

1/4 cup almond milk

1 1/2 tsp. minced garlic

1 tsp. minced fresh parsley

1/2 tsp. fresh lemon juice

Pinch of salt

Combine all ingredients in a glass jar with a tight fitting lid and shake to combine or use a whisk. Store at room temperature and shake before using.

## Creamy Basil Balsamic Vinaigrette

1 Tbsp. balsamic vinegar

2 Tbsp. olive oil

1/2 tsp. dried basil

1/2 tsp. onion powder

1/8 tsp. sea salt or Herbamare

4 drops liquid stevia or 1 tsp. honey or agave

2 Tbsp. coconut milk

Combine all ingredients in a glass jar with a tight fitting lid and shake to combine or use a whisk. Store in the refrigerator and shake before using. Makes 1/2 cup.

## Sweet Ginger Dressing

2 Tbsp. white miso

1 Tbsp. fresh ginger

1 tsp. sesame oil, toasted

1 Tbsp. mild oil, such as sunflower or avocado

2 Tbsp. agave or honey

1 Tbsp. water

1 tsp. apple cider vinegar

Combine all ingredients in a high speed blender or food processor and blend until smooth. Store in the refrigerator.

This dressing goes well on salads containing sea vegetables, cucumbers, etc...

# Salads

## Tomato Feta Salad

4 medium tomatoes

1/2 cup thinly sliced red onion

1/2 red bell pepper, cut into thin strips

1/2 yellow or orange bell pepper, cut into thin strips

1 small cucumber, sliced

1/2 tsp. dried marjoram

1 cup black olives

1/3 cup olive oil

1/4 cup red wine vinegar

1/2 lb. feta cheese

Cut the tomatoes into 1 inch chunks.  Combine all ingredients in a bowl and toss gently.  Let marinate an hour or so before serving. Serves 4-6

---

## Summer Squash Salad

2 cups thinly sliced zucchini

2 cups yellow squash, thinly sliced

1/2 cup freshly grated Parmesan cheese

1/4 cup apple cider vinegar

1/4 tsp. sea salt

1/4 tsp. pepper

1/2 tsp. dried basil leaves

2 Tbsp. olive oil

1 tsp. minced garlic

1/2 cup red onion, thinly sliced

2 tomatoes, cut into wedges

In a large bowl, stir together the cheese, vinegar, salt, pepper, basil, oil, and garlic.  Add the other vegetables and toss to coat.  Serve or let marinate.  Serves 4-6

# Shrimp Salad

1 medium jicama, cut into matchsticks

1 ripe mango, cut into short strips

2 cups cooked wildcaught shrimp

1 ripe avocado, cut into small chunks

1 Tbsp. sweet onion, minced

### Dressing:

1 jalepeno pepper, seeded and chopped

1 bunch cilantro

1 large lime

Blend dressing ingredients together and pour over other ingredients in a glass bowl. Season to taste and serve immediately.

Serves 4

---

# Marinated Greens

1 bunch of kale or collards

1 red bell pepper, chopped

1/4 cup red onion, very thinly sliced

### Dressing:

1 Tbsp. tamari sauce

1 Tbsp. lemon juice

2 Tbsp. olive oil

1 tsp. honey or other sweetener

1 Tbsp. sesame seeds

Tear or slice the kale into small, bite-sized pieces and place in a bowl with the bell pepper and onion. Mix the dressing ingredients in a container, except for the sesame seeds. Pour the dressing over the greens and stir to coat well. Sprinkle with sesame seeds and let marinate for a few hours before serving. Keeps well for several days in the refrigerator. Note: This is also good with 1/2 cup of kimchi mixed into it.

# My Favorite Salad

2 handfuls of spring mix lettuce or baby spinach

1/3 of a red onion, cut into thin rings

1 ripe tomato, chopped, or 1/2 cup cherry tomatoes

1 ripe avocado, peeled and chopped

1/8 cup raisins or dried cranberries

1/8 cup walnuts or pecans

Basil Vinaigrette from page 111

Place all ingredients in a bowl and add the dressing. Serve immediately.

Serves 1-2

# Asian Salad

1 napa cabbage, cut into thin strips

2 carrots, shredded

3-4 green onions, chopped

1/2 cup grated diakon radish

1 red bell pepper, cut into thin strips

1/2-1 cup sliced mushrooms

1 cup mung bean sprouts

Asian Ginger Dressing (page 112 or Sweet Ginger Dressing on page 114 )

Place all the vegetables in a salad bowl and top with the dressing. Serve immediately

Serves 3-4

## Quinoa Salad

1 1/2 cups quinoa, soaked in water overnight or for several hours, then rinsed and drained until water runs clear

1 Tbsp. olive oil

1 onion, chopped

2 cloves garlic, peeled and chopped

1 1/2 cups water or broth

1 tsp. cumin

1/8 tsp. cayenne pepper

1/2 tsp. sea salt

1/2 cup chopped red bell pepper

1/4-1/2 cup chopped fresh cilantro

1/4 cup chopped cherry tomatoes (optional)

1/2 cup cubed cooked chicken or other meat (optional)

1 Tbsp. olive oil

Sea salt to taste

Heat oil in a large skillet and stir in onion and cook until it begins to turn translucent. Add garlic and cook for another minute. Add quinoa to the pan and add just enough water or broth to cover the grains. Stir in the cumin, cayenne, and salt. Bring the mixture to a boil, cover, reduce heat and simmer for 20 minutes.

Remove cooked quinoa from pan and place into a bowl and let cool. Add the remaining ingredients and stir to combine. Taste and adjust seasonings.

Serves 3-4

# Greek Salad

2 tsp. fresh lemon juice

2 tsp. red wine vinegar

2 Tbsp. olive oil

1/4 tsp. oregano, dried

Sea salt and pepper

1 large ripe tomato, cut into chunks

1/2 cucumber, peeled and chopped

1/4 medium red onion, thinly sliced

10 large leaves of romaine lettuce hearts

16 large mint leaves, optional

5 oz. feta cheese, cut into 3/4 inch cubes, optional

1/2 cup black olives

In a small jar or bowl, mix the first 5 ingredients. Put the tomato, cucumber, and onion in a salad bowl and sprinkle with some sea salt. Then pour about 1 Tbsp. of the vinaigrette over the vegetables and toss lightly. Cut the lettuce leaves into bite sized pieces, and cut the mint into thin strips. Add the lettuce to the salad bowl. Add one cube of feta to the remaining dressing and mash with a fork. Pour over the lettuce and vegetables and toss. Add the feta and olives and toss gently. Serves 2-3.

---

# Cucumber and Pumpkin Seed Salad

2 large cucumbers, peeled and sliced

3 Tbsp. pumpkin seeds

1/2 cup raw macadamia nuts

2 Tbsp. white miso

1 tsp. turmeric

1 clove garlic

2 Tbsp. lemon juice

Blend the nuts with 1 cup filtered water, miso, turmeric, garlic, lemon juice, and salt. Toss with the cucumbers and pumpkin seeds and season to taste with the salt. Serves 2

# Shrimp Salad Wrap

1 cup precooked wildcaught salad shrimp

2 green onions, chopped

1 carrot, shredded

1/2 zucchini, grated

1/2 cup chopped cilantro

1 avocado

1/2 tsp. lemon juice

1 1/2 tsp. red wine vinegar or apple cider vinegar

1 tsp. honey or agave

1/4 tsp. Old Bay seasoning

1 Tbsp. olive oil

Sea salt to taste

3-4 large romaine lettuce leaves or gluten free tortillas

In a bowl, mix the first 5 ingredients. Mash the avocado and add the lemon juice and some sea salt. In another jar or bowl, combine the vinegar, honey, Old Bay, olive oil, and some salt. Pour this dressing over the shrimp and vegetables and stir well.

To serve, spread a couple of tablespoons of the avocado mixture down the center rib of the inside of the lettuce leaf. Top it with the shrimp mixture. Fill all lettuce leaves or tortillas the same way and serve like soft tacos. Serves 1-2

---

# Broccoli Salad

2 bunches of broccoli, chopped

2 cups red seedless grapes

1 cup raisins

1 cup roasted pecans

1/2 cup diced red onion

### Dressing:

3/4 cup mayonnaise

3/4 cup plain yogurt or Kefir Sauce

3 Tbsp. honey or agave

1 Tbsp. apple cider vinegar

Pinch of salt

Toss salad mixture with the dressing and serve chilled. Serves 10

# Chicken Salad

A simple and delicious chicken salad can be as easy as taking leftover chicken and chopping it up and then adding some chopped mild onion, carrot, avocado, and sunflower sprouts. Put it in a bowl and add some mayonnaise (page 113 ). Serve it on a bed of salad greens.

**Variation:** mix 2 Tbsp. mayonnaise with 1/4 cup plain yogurt or coconut milk, 4 tsp. fresh lemon juice, and 1 tsp. honey. Add diced chicken and some halved grapes, a diced apple, a diced pear, and 1 cup pecans and toss it all together. Season to taste with sea salt.

---

# Black Bean Salad

2 cups black beans, cooked

1 cup frozen corn, thawed

1/2 red bell pepper, finely chopped

3 green onions, finely chopped

1 large carrot, thinly sliced

1/2 cup chopped fresh cilantro (optional)

1/4 cup pumpkin seeds (optional)

### Dressing:

2 tsp. apple cider vinegar

1/2 cup mild oil (avocado, grapeseed, etc..)

1 tsp. garlic powder

1 tsp. sea salt

A pinch or more of ground cayenne pepper

1-2 tsp. agave nectar (to taste)

In a salad bowl, combine all the vegetable ingredients. Place the dressing ingredients in a small jar and shake to combine or mix together in a small bowl. Pour the dressing over the salad and stir to coat with the dressing. Taste and adjust seasonings if necessary.

## Blender Salad

*This is a great way to consume more green vegetables. It can be pre-pared once a week. Adapted from the* Great Cleanse Lifestyle Journal.

2 cucumbers, peeled

3 cloves garlic

1 inch fresh ginger root

6 stalks celery

1 cup lemon or lime juice

Blend these ingredients until liquefied. Then add the following ingredients:

   16 oz. spinach

   1 cup sprouts

   2 avocados

   1/2 bunch cilantro

   1/2 bunch basil

   1/2 bunch parsley

   1-2 tsp. sea salt

   1/8 tsp. cayenne pepper

   Add enough water to allow blender to liquefy the contents, leaving 1 inch of air space at the top of the blender. Blend until smooth. Pour into glass jars and refrigerate. This will keep fresh for up to a week. Makes about 7 pints. Dilute with water if needed.

# Fermented Vegetables

## Kimchi (Korean Sauerkraut)

1 Nappa cabbage, cored and finely shredded

1 bunch green onions, chopped

1 cup carrots, grated

1 cup daikon radish, grated

1 Tbsp. freshly grated gingerroot

3 cloves garlic, minced

1/2 tsp. dried red chili flakes

1 Tbsp. sea salt or to taste

Mix all the ingredients together in a large bowl. Taste to adjust salt. It should taste lightly salted. Place into a fermenting crock or a wide mouth glass jar. Pack down each layer as you fill the container with the vegetables. Make sure to leave a few inches at the top of the container for an airspace. The vegetables will bubble and expand as they ferment.

If you are using the jar method, once the jar is packed, place a few large leaves of cabbage on top to hold down the small bits of vegetables. Then place a smaller glass jar inside the large jar to hold down the cabbage leaves so they stay submerged in the brine that will form. A baby food jar works really well for this. Then put the lid on the large jar so that when tightened, the baby food jar compresses the vegetables. This will allow you to watch the fermentation process. As the bubbles form and the brine rises, you can crack the large jar's lid to allow any air that has built up to escape.

Keep at 68 degrees for 2-4 weeks. Every few days, check it and slightly unscrew the lid to release any air that has built up. When it stops bubbling, it is ready to be put into the refrigerator. You can eat it at this point, or let it age further in the refrigerator. It will keep several months in the refrigerator. Make sure the vegetables stay submerged in the brine so that mold doesn't form.

Makes 1/2 gallon.

## Sauerkraut

3 large heads of organic cabbage
Sea salt

Cut the cabbage into quarters and cut out the center core. Slice very thinly using a knife, mandolin, or a food processor blade.

Place in a large bowl. Sprinkle with sea salt and stir well to combine. Taste some of the cabbage to test saltiness. It should taste lightly salted.

Place into a fermenting crock or a wide mouth glass jar. Pack down each layer as you fill the container with the cabbage. Make sure to leave a few inches at the top of the container for an airspace. The vegetable juice/brine will produce bubbles and expand as it ferments.

If you are using the jar method, once the jar is packed, place a few large leaves of cabbage on top to hold down the small bits of cabbage. Then place a smaller glass jar inside the large jar to hold down the cabbage leaves so they stay submerged in the brine that will form. A baby food jar works really well for this. Then put the lid on the large jar so that when tightened, the baby food jar compresses the vegetables. This will allow you to watch the fermentation process. As the bubbles form and the brine rises, you can crack the large jar's lid to allow any air that has built up to escape.

Keep at 68 degrees for 2-4 weeks. Every few days, check it and slightly unscrew the lid to release any air that has built up. When it stops bubbling, it is ready to be put into the refrigerator. You can eat it at this point, or let it age further in the refrigerator. It will keep several months in the refrigerator. Make sure the vegetables stay submerged in the brine so that mold doesn't form.

Makes 1/2 gallon.

# Sauerkraut Apple Salad

3 cups Sauerkraut

1 tart apple, chopped

1 small onion, chopped

3/4 cup chopped dill pickle

3 Tbsp. lemon juice

1 Tbsp. honey or agave

1 Tbsp. dried basil

1 Tbsp. dill weed

1 tsp. sea salt

1/4 cup oil, such as sunflower or avocado oil

Combine all ingredients in a bowl.  Cover and refrigerate for at least 2 hours before serving.

Serves 4-6

# Sauces

## Nacho Sauce

1 large red bell pepper

1/2 cup raw cashews or almonds (or almond butter)

2 Tbsp. tahini (or ground sesame seeds)

2 Tbsp. nutritional yeast

1-1 1/2 tsp. sea salt

2 tsp. onion powder

1 tsp. garlic powder

Juice of 1 lemon juice

1/8 tsp. cayenne powder or to taste


Blend all ingredients until smooth and creamy. Add water to thin if necessary. Store in refrigerator. It will thicken up in the refrigerator. This can be used as a dip.

---

## Kefir Sauce (Dairy free)

*This delicious sauce is a great non-dairy substitute for sour cream!*

2 cups raw macadamia nuts

1 packet kefir starter culture


Soak the nuts in water to cover for 1-2 hours. Drain and rinse. Blend with 2—2 1/2 cups of water until completely smooth. Place in a glass jar and add the kefir starter. Put a lid on loosely and let sit at room temperature for 12-24 hours, depending on the level of sourness you desire. Loosen the lid as you see the bubbles form in the mixture to allow any built up pressure to escape.

When it is done, stir it and store in the refrigerator. Keeps 2 weeks.

Makes 1 quart.

# Sun-Dried Tomato Sauce

1 jar of sun-dried tomatoes with herbs

1 large tomato

1 large red bell pepper

Sea salt or Italian herbal seasoning to taste

Combine all ingredients in a food processor and mix until thick and chunky. This makes a great topping for broiled salmon or any other meats. Can be used as a filling to stuff avocados too.

# Alfredo Sauce

1 cup macadamia nuts (soak in water for 1 hour for easier blending)

1 cup water

2 Tbsp. olive oil

Juice of 1 lemon

2 cloves of garlic

Dash of Dijon mustard or dry mustard

Sea salt to taste

Blend all ingredients until smooth in a high speed blender or food processor. Taste and adjust seasonings.

This is very nice served over zucchini peeled into strips to resemble noodles, topped with tomatoes, bell pepper, avocado, and chicken.

# Red Bell Pepper Sauce

2 red bell peppers

1/2 cup lemon juice

1 cup macadamia nuts

2 tsp. soy sauce

2 cloves garlic

Blend all ingredients until smooth in a high speed blender or food processor. Taste and adjust seasoning.

# Mushroom Gravy

2 cups portabello mushrooms

3-4 Tbsp. miso

1 Tbsp. filtered water

1/4 tsp. garlic powder

1/2 tsp. thyme

Blend all ingredients until smooth in a high speed blender or food processor. Taste and adjust seasonings.

This is very nice served over steamed cauliflower, potatoes, etc...

---

# Cranberry Relish

4 cups raw cranberries, washed

1 orange, peel left on, quartered and seeded

1/4 cup candied ginger

2 Tbsp. maple syrup or agave

1/2 cup toasted walnuts or pecans, optional

In a food processor, combine 2 cups of the cranberries and half of the orange. Process until finely chopped. Add the remaining ingredients aside from the nuts and process to a fine consistency. Stir in the nuts if desired. Chill before serving.

# Side Dishes

# Braised Vegetables

This technique involves sautéing some vegetables first, then adding a small amount of liquid to the pan and simmering it until the vegetables are finished cooking. It makes an easy and delicious side dish.

## Quick-Braised Vegetables

1 pound of vegetables (green beans, carrots, asparagus, etc...)

1 Tbsp. olive oil

1 Tbsp. butter

1/2 tsp. sea salt

1/3 cup chicken broth

1 tsp. Dijon mustard (optional)

Wash and trim vegetables, cutting carrots into strips , if using them. Heat the olive oil and 2 tsp butter in a 10-12 inch skillet on the stove on medium-high heat. Make sure the pan you use has a lid. Add the vegetables to the pan so they are in a single layer. Cook without stirring for about 3-4 minutes. Toss and turn them and cook for another 2 minutes. Pour the chicken broth into the pan and immediately put the lid on the pan. Reduce the heat so that the broth is just simmering. Cook for 3-5 minutes or until the vegetables are cooked. Remove from the heat and add the optional Dijon mustard, and remaining butter and toss to combine. Season to taste. Serve immediately.
Serves 2-3

## Braised Greens

1 large onion or 1 leek, sliced

2 bunches of greens (kale, collards, mustard greens, beet greens, etc..) washed and torn into bite sized pieces

1/2 cup chicken broth

Sea salt to taste

In a large skillet, heat 2 Tbsp. oil over medium heat and add the onion or leek. Cook until it softens. Add the greens and pour the stock into the pan. Cover and cook on medium low heat for 15-25 minutes or until greens are tender. Season to taste with sea salt.

# Braised Zucchini with Rosemary

1 Tbsp. butter, olive oil, or coconut oil

1 onion, thinly sliced

1 clove garlic, minced

4 medium zucchini, sliced

1/2 tsp. dried rosemary, or 1 tsp. fresh rosemary

1 tomato, chopped

1/2 cup chicken stock

2-3 Tbsp. freshly grated Parmesan cheese (optional)

Heat the butter in a large skillet and sauté the onion and garlic for about 5 minutes. Add the zucchini and rosemary and sauté for 3-5 minutes. Add the tomato and broth, cover, reduce the heat and cook for 10 minutes. Add the salt to taste and sprinkle with Parmesan cheese if desired. Serves 4-5

---

# Zucchini with Basil

3 medium zucchini, sliced 1/4 inch thick

2 Tbsp olive oil

1 tsp. garlic powder

1 tsp. dried basil (optional)

2 tsp. red wine vinegar or balsamic vinegar (optional)

Place the sliced zucchini in a large bowl and add the olive oil, stirring to coat all the zucchini. Then add the garlic powder, stirring to coat. Place the zucchini on a broiling pan in a single layer. Broil 4-5 inches from the heat source for about 5-6 minutes, or until they start to get golden speckles. Turn off the heat and shut oven door so they can continue to cook from the warmth of the oven a few more minutes. Remove and place them in a serving dish. Sprinkle with sea salt or Herbamare and sprinkle with the optional herbs and vinegar. Let marinate a few minutes before serving. Serves 2-3

## Vegetables with Lemon Butter

*This is a quick and easy way to make a delicious side dish that goes with just about any meal.*

2 cups water

2 cups vegetables, such as sugar snap peas, broccoli, green beans, or asparagus

1 Tbsp. butter or mild tasting oil, such as avocado oil

1/2 Tbsp. fresh lemon juice

1/2 tsp. dried tarragon leaves

1/4 tsp. onion powder

Bring the water to a boil in a saucepan. While the water heats, prepare the vegetables: snap the peas, or cut the broccoli into bite sized pieces. Place the vegetables into the boiling water and let cook for 2-3 minutes, then pour them into a colander to let drain.

Mix the butter or oil and remaining ingredients in the hot saucepan to melt the butter and to combine the ingredients. Add the cooked vegetables to the saucepan and stir to coat them with the mixture. Season with sea salt. Serve immediately. Serves 2-4

---

## Broiled Eggplant

3-4 long, thin Chinese eggplant

3-4 Tbsp. olive oil

1/2 tsp. garlic powder, optional

Slice the eggplant into 1/4 inch slices. Coat both sides of the eggplant with olive oil and sprinkle with garlic powder. Place on a baking sheet or broiler pan. Broil 4 inches from the heat source until the eggplant starts to get brown speckles.

Remove from oven and turn them over. Place back under broiler and cook 5-7 minutes. Season to taste with sea salt and serve immediately. Serves 2-3

## Sweet Potatoes

2-3 sweet potatoes, peeled and sliced into 1/4 inch slices

2-3 Tbsp. coconut oil

1/2 tsp. cinnamon

Sea salt

Preheat the oven to 350 degrees. Coat the sliced potatoes with the coconut oil and spread out on a baking sheet. Sprinkle with cinnamon. Bake for 35 –45 minutes or until done. Season to taste with salt.

Serves 4-6

---

## Marinated Mushrooms

1 1/2 Tbsp. red wine vinegar

1/3 cup olive oil

1 tsp. onion powder

1/2 tsp. sea salt

1 Tbsp. fresh parsley, chopped

1 tsp. dry mustard powder or Dijon mustard

2 tsp. honey or agave

1/2 tsp. garlic powder

1/2 lb. mushrooms, cut up if large

1/2 sweet onion, thinly sliced

1/2 red bell pepper, thinly sliced

Combine all ingredients except the mushrooms in a bowl. Add the mushrooms and stir well to coat. Let marinate for several hours.

Serves 2

# Pesto stuffed Mushrooms or Tomatoes

1 large bunch basil, coarsely chopped

1/4 cup lemon juice

3 cloves garlic, chopped

2 cups walnuts

3/4 tsp. sea salt

1/4 cup olive oil

20 button mushrooms or portabello mushrooms or sliced tomatoes

2 Tbsp. tamari

2 Tbsp. olive oil

Mix the tamari and 2 Tbsp. olive oil in a shallow dish and add the mushrooms, stirring to coat. Let marinate while you fix the pesto.

Combine the basil, lemon juice, garlic, walnuts, sea salt, and oil in a food processor and process to a thick paste. Fill the mushroom caps with the pesto or spread on top of sliced tomatoes. The mushrooms can be warmed in the oven on the lowest setting or in a dehydrator.
Serves 4

---

# Roasted Beets, Carrots, and Parsnips

6 large beets, peeled and quartered

5 parsnips, peeled and cut into large chunks

5 large carrots, cut into large chunks

2-3 Tbsp. olive oil

Preheat the oven to 350 degrees. Place all of the vegetables into a large bowl. Drizzle 2-3 Tbsp. olive oil on them and stir to coat them with the oil. Lay them out on a baking sheet in a single layer and sprinkle them with sea salt. Place in the oven and let cook for 1 1/2 hours or until cooked to your liking.

Serves 4

# Mexican Rice and Beans

2 cups cooked brown rice

1 1/2 cups salsa, drained

2 cups cooked black beans

2 tsp. ground cumin

1 tsp. chili powder

1/4 cup finely chopped fresh cilantro

Combine all ingredients and season to taste with sea salt.

Serves 3-4

# Zucchini and Onions

3-4 zucchini, sliced

1 red onion, cut into slices

2 Tbsp. olive oil

Sea salt

Place the vegetables in a large bowl and coat with the olive oil. Spread the vegetables out on a broiling pan in a single layer and sprinkle with salt. Broil until the vegetables start to get browned. Turn off broiler, but leave the vegetables in the oven for a few minutes to continue to cook. Remove from oven and season to taste. Serve immediately. Serves 2

# Stuffed Avocados

3 avocados

Sun-dried Tomato Sauce page 127

Sea salt to taste

Cut avocados in half and remove seed. Using a large spoon, scoop out the meat of the avocados. Fill the avocado halves with the Tomato Sauce. Serves 3-4

## Vegetables with Sun-Dried Tomatoes

*A delicious and easy side dish for any meal!*

1 lb. vegetables (asparagus, green beans, sugar snap peas, etc..)

1/4 cup thinly sliced red onion

1/4 cup sun-dried tomatoes in oil, thinly sliced or chopped

1 tsp. balsamic vinegar

1/2 tsp. garlic powder

2 Tbsp. olive oil

Bring a pot of water to a boil.  Put vegetables in the boiling water and let cook for 2-3 minutes.  Remove them and put them in a bowl or serving dish.  Combine remaining ingredients and add to vegetables, stirring to coat.  Season to taste with sea salt and serve immediately.  Serves 2-3

## Grilled Zucchini

1/2 cup olive oil

2 Tbsp. chopped fresh herbs, such as oregano, thyme, rosemary, basil, or a mixture of several herbs

4 cloves garlic, minced

1/4 tsp. crushed red pepper

6 medium zucchini or yellow squash, cut into large pieces (1-1 1/2 inch)

Freshly grated Parmesan cheese, optional

Prepare the grill.  Combine the oil, herbs, garlic, and red pepper in a dish.  Add the vegetables and stir to coat.  Let sit to marinate for a few minutes.  Thread them on a skewer and place on the grill.  Cook for 5 minutes on one side, turn over, and grill for 10 more minutes or until they are tender and starting to brown.  Serve immediately, sprinkled with the cheese and sea salt.  Serves 4

Note:  This can also be made with other vegetables

# Roasted Vegetables

1 lb. any vegetable (squash, potatoes, carrots, green beans, etc..)

2-3 Tbsp. olive oil

1/2 tsp. sea salt

1/2 tsp. garlic powder, optional

1/2 tsp. thyme or rosemary, optional

Preheat oven to 400 degrees. Prepare the vegetables by cutting them into 3/4 inch to 1 inch pieces. Toss the vegetable with the oil to coat and the salt (and optional garlic and/or herbs). Place on a roasting pan or broiler pan so that they do not overlap each other. Roast in the oven for 30-45 minutes, or until they start to brown, stirring once halfway through the cooking time. Season to taste and serve warm or at room temperature. Serves 2-3

# Asparagus

1 bunch asparagus

1-2 Tbsp olive oil

1/4 tsp. garlic powder

Wash asparagus and pat dry. Snap off the bottom inch or two of the stem that is too tough to eat. Coat them with the oil and sprinkle with the garlic powder. Place on a broiling pan and broil 4 inches from the heating element for 8-10 minutes or until they start to brown slightly, stirring once halfway through cooking time. Sprinkle with salt and serve immediately. Serves 2-3

## Easy Rice

2 Tbsp. butter, coconut oil, or olive oil

1 cup finely chopped onion

2 cups brown rice

3 cups chicken broth

2 Tbsp. minced green onion, optional

2 Tbsp. minced green parsley, optional

2 garlic cloves, minced, optional

Preheat oven to 350 degrees. Heat oil in a large oven-proof saucepan over medium heat. Add the onion and sauté for 5 minutes. Add the rice, broth, and remaining optional ingredients if using. Bring to a boil. Cover end place pot in the oven and bake until liquid is absorbed and rice is tender, about 45 minutes. Serves 6-8

---

## Quinoa

2 cups quinoa, soaked in water for several hours, and then rinsed and drained until water runs clear

1 bunch green onions, chopped

2 Tbsp. olive oil

1/2 tsp. sea salt

3 cloves garlic, minced

3-4 cups broth

1 tsp. sea salt

In a large skillet, sauté the onions in the oil for a few minutes. Add the garlic and sauté for another minutes. Add the quinoa and broth (the broth should just barely cover the quinoa), and salt. Bring to a boil, reduce heat, cover, and let simmer for 20-25 minutes on low heat. Serves 4-6

## Vegetables with Cumin

2 Tbsp. olive oil or coconut oil

1 onion, chopped

1 red bell pepper, chopped

1 zucchini, quartered and sliced

1 tsp. cumin

1 large pinch red pepper flakes

1 tsp. salt

2 tomatoes, chopped

1/4 cup broth or white wine

2 Tbsp. fresh parsley, finely chopped

In a large skillet, heat the oil over medium heat. Saute the onion, pepper, and zucchini in the oil for 6-10 minutes. Add the cumin, red pepper flakes, salt, and tomatoes, and cook another 5 minutes. Add broth or wine and cook until most of the liquid is evaporated and the vegetables are tender. Serves 3-4

## Red Smashed Potatoes

1 lb. small red potatoes

2 cloves garlic

1 bay leaf

1 Tbsp. sea salt

2 Tbsp. butter or olive oil

1/4 cup almond milk

2 Tbsp. fresh parsley, chopped

Cut potatoes in half and place in a 3 quart saucepan. Fill saucepan with water to cover the potatoes by an inch. Add garlic, bay leaves, and salt to the water and bring to a boil. Reduce heat and simmer for 20 minutes. Drain and discard garlic and bay leaf. Put potatoes back into saucepan and add butter, almond milk, and more salt to taste. Lightly smash the potatoes and mix in parsley. Serves 4

## Beans from Scratch

*Here is an easy way to cook dried beans.*

2 cups dried beans, soaked overnight in water to cover

1 onion, cut in half

2-3 cloves garlic

2 carrots, optional

2 celery stalks, optional

1 tsp. dried thyme, optional

2-3 bay leaves

Drain beans in a colander after soaking overnight. Place in a large pot and add onion, garlic, carrots, celery, thyme, and bay leaves. Add enough filtered water to cover beans by an inch. Bring to a boil, then reduce heat and let simmer for about 1 hour.

Test the beans to see if they are cooked by removing 5 beans from the pot and eating them. If they are not all done, continue to cook 15 more minutes, then repeat test.

When beans are cooked, add 2 Tbsp. or more of sea salt to the bean water and let them soak it up for 15 minutes. Discard the vegetables and bay leaves before using the beans. Makes 5-6 cups.

---

## Broccoli

*A deliciously simple way to season steamed broccoli.*

1 head of broccoli, steamed until just tender, about 7-9 minutes

1/2 tsp. garlic powder

2 tsp. onion powder

1 small lemon wedge, about 1/4 of a lemon

1 Tbsp. olive oil (or basil or tarragon infused olive oil)

Put the steamed, hot broccoli in a bowl, and add the remaining ingredients. Toss gently to coat and season to taste with sea salt. Serve immediately. Serves 2-4

## Butternut Squash with Apples and Cranberries

1 butternut squash

3 apples

1/2 cup dried cranberries

2 Tbsp. unrefined sugar or agave

1/2 tsp. sea salt

2 Tbsp. melted coconut oil

Preheat oven to 400 degrees. Peel, seed, and cut the squash and apples into cubes and put in a casserole dish with the cranberries.

Pour the melted coconut oil over the squash and apples and sprinkle with the sweetener and salt. Toss well to coat.

Cover dish and bake 45 minutes to 1 hour, or until the squash is tender, stirring once halfway through the baking time. Serves 4-6

---

## Roasted Potatoes with Garlic and Rosemary

2 lbs. red potatoes

2 Tbsp. olive oil

1 tsp. garlic powder

2 tsp. fresh rosemary, minced

Wash and cut potatoes in half, then in half again, so they are evenly sized. Place in a bowl and drizzle the olive oil over them, add the seasonings and stir to coat well. Place on a single layer on a baking sheet and cook at 400 degrees for 30-45 minutes or until starting to brown. When done, season to taste with sea salt. Serves 3

# Ratatouille

4 Tbsp. olive oil

4 cloves garlic, minced

1 Tbsp. fresh parsley, chopped

1 eggplant, cut into 1/2 inch cubes

1/2 cup grated Parmesan cheese, optional

2 zucchini, cut into 1/2 inch cubes

1 onion, cut into 1/2 inch cubes

1 red bell pepper, cut into 1/2 inch cubes

1 cup cherry tomatoes, cut in half

Preheat oven to 350 degrees.  Heat 2 Tbsp. of olive oil in a large skillet over medium heat.  Add the garlic and sauté for a couple of minutes.  Add the parsley and the eggplant.  Saute until the eggplant starts to soften, about 10 minutes.

Meanwhile, place the other vegetables on a large baking sheet and drizzle with the remaining olive oil.  Stir gently to coat.  Add the cooked eggplant to the vegetables on the baking sheet.  Sprinkle the vegetables with sea salt and parmesan cheese if desired.

Bake for 45-60 minutes.   Serves 4-6

# Baby Bok Choy Braise

2 baby bok choy, coarsely chopped

2 Tbsp. olive oil

1 onion, chopped

1 clove garlic, minced

1/4 tsp. minced gingerroot

1/4 cup chicken or turkey broth

Heat a large skillet over medium heat.  Add the olive oil and the onion and cook until it softens, about 7-10 minutes.  Add the remaining ingredients, cover, and reduce heat to medium-low, so it slightly simmers.  Cook for 15-20 minutes.  Season to taste with sea salt or tamari.

# Main
# Dish

## Roast Chicken

1 whole chicken, giblets removed from inside cavity

1/2 lemon

4 cloves garlic

Small handful of parsley

1 tsp. dried thyme

Optional: 2-3 cups of other vegetables cut into large 1 inch chunks (onion, potatoes, carrots, zucchini, sweet potato, winter squash, etc..) to roast along with the chicken.

Preheat the oven to 350 degrees. Rinse the chicken with cold water and pat dry with paper towels. Place the chicken in a large roasting pan and put the lemon, garlic, and parsley inside the cavity of the chicken. Sprinkle outside of chicken with the thyme and sea salt.

If you want to roast some vegetables along with the chicken, coat them with some olive oil and add them to the pan. Just scatter them around the chicken in a single layer. Now place the pan in the oven and cook for about 20 minutes per pound of chicken. Serve with a green salad and the vegetables for an easy meal.

---

## Broiled Fish Fillets

Fish fillets ( flounder, salmon, snapper, etc...), 1 per person

2 Tbsp. melted coconut oil

1/2-1 tsp. Old Bay Seasoning

Pat the fish completely dry with paper towels. Place on a broiling pan and coat with the oil on both sides. Sprinkle lightly with Herbamare and Old Bay. Place pan on a rack in the oven so it is about 4 inches from the heating element at the top of the oven. Broil on high until the fish turns opaque and just starts to release it's juices around the edges. It should be done quickly, in about 5-8 minutes. Remove it from the oven to check doneness by inserting a fork into the fish and twisting the fork. If the fish meat separates easily, it is done cooking.

# Pasta with Marinara Sauce

3-4 zucchini, peeled

**Sauce:**  2 1/2 cups tomatoes

10 sun-dried tomatoes, soaked in water for 1-2 hours

3 dates or 1/4 cup raisins, soaked in water 1 hour

1/4 cup olive oil

1 tsp. garlic powder

2 Tbsp. fresh parsley

1 tsp. sea salt

**Optional toppings:** Marinated Mushroom recipe on page 133 or the Pesto on page 134.

To make the pasta, run a vegetable peeler lengthwise down each zucchini to make ribbons. Continue peeling all the way around them until you get to the center seeds. Place them in a bowl and toss with a teaspoon of salt and a couple tablespoons of olive oil.

For the sauce, place all of the sauce ingredients in a food processor and blend until smooth. It should be thick. Place this over the zucchini pasta. Can be served like this or you can add the Marinated Mushrooms and vegetables to the tomato sauce.   Serves 2

# Turkey Burgers

2 lbs. ground turkey

1 medium sweet onion, minced

1 large handful of spinach leaves, diced

1/2  cup ground flaxseeds

1/2 tsp. sea salt

1/4 tsp. ground pepper

1/2 tsp. garlic powder

1/4 tsp. cumin powder

2 dashes hot sauce

Mix all ingredients and form into patties. Cook in a skillet on medium heat on the stove or cook on a grill. Serves 4-6

# Spaghetti

2 Tbsp. butter or olive oil

1 onion, chopped

2 cloves garlic, minced

1 carrot, thinly sliced

1/2 cup sliced mushrooms, optional

1 zucchini, cut in half and sliced thinly into half moons

1 lb. ground meat (turkey, beef, venison, or buffalo)

1 Tbsp. fresh basil or 1 Tbsp. pesto

1 28 oz. can of tomatoes, chopped (or fresh tomatoes)

1 small can of tomato paste

Pinch of cinnamon or a teaspoon of honey

Pasta, spaghetti squash, or zucchini peeled into ribbons

Melt the butter in a large skillet. Add the onion and sauté for a few minutes. Add the other vegetables and continue to cook until they are almost done. Add the meat and cook for a few minutes. Add the tomatoes, basil, tomato paste, and let simmer for 15-20 minutes. Add salt to taste and the cinnamon or honey. Serve over pasta and sprinkle with freshly grated parmesan cheese if desired.   Serves 2-3

---

# Skip's Chicken

*This delicious chicken recipe can be cooked on the stovetop or in a crockpot on the lowest setting.  The meat becomes so tender that it falls off the bone.*

Chicken thighs with skin, (1-2 per person)

Tamari or soy sauce

Garlic powder

In a large  cast iron skillet or other heavy bottomed skillet, place the chicken in the pan and sprinkle each chicken thigh with about a teaspoon of the tamari. Then sprinkle about  1/4 tsp. of the garlic powder on each thigh. Cover the skillet and cook on the lowest possible setting on top of the stove. Let cook for 4-5 hours or more, turning the chicken over half way through the process.

# Fajitas

## Marinade:

> 3 Tbsp. olive oil
>
> 2 tsp. fresh lime juice
>
> 2 tsp. minced fresh garlic
>
> 1 tsp. ground cumin
>
> 1/2 tsp. sea salt

1 1/2 lbs. steak or chicken cut into thin strips

3 onions, sliced

2 bell peppers, sliced

2 cups romaine lettuce, thinly sliced

1 cup chopped tomatoes or salsa

6 green onions, sliced

Other optional toppings: Kefir sauce (page 126), guacamole, cilantro, or chopped avocado

Whole grain tortillas or lettuce (for a fajita salad)

Combine all marinade ingredients in a large dish or bowl. Add the meat and mix well. Let marinate 30 minutes or up to 24 hours (in refrigerator).

In a large skillet, heat 2 Tbsp. of coconut or olive oil over medium heat and add the sliced onions and cook for 5-7 minutes, then add the bell pepper and continue cooking until softened. Remove from pan and add the meat. Cook, stirring often, until done. Serve meat in the tortillas or over a bed of lettuce. Top with remaining ingredients.

Serves 4

# Tacos

1 lb. ground meat (turkey, beef, venison, or buffalo)

1 onion, chopped

2 cloves garlic, minced

1/2 cup salsa

2 tsp. chili powder

1/2 tsp. cumin

2 cups romaine lettuce, thinly sliced

1/2 cup chopped green onion

1 cup chopped tomatoes

1 cup shredded raw cheese, optional

1/2 cup Kefir sauce (page 126), optional

Taco shells or lettuce

In a large skillet, cook the meat with the onion and garlic until cooked through. Drain off excess fat. Stir in the salsa, chili powder, cumin, and 1/4 tsp. of salt. Fill taco shells with the meat mixture and top with additional toppings. Or serve the meat over lettuce and top with the toppings and crumbled corn chips. Serves 4.

---

# Tarragon Chicken

2 lbs. chicken thighs with skin on

2 Tbsp. Dijon mustard

2 Tbsp. melted butter or coconut oil

1 Tbsp. dried tarragon leaves (or 3 Tbsp. fresh tarragon leaves)

Preheat oven to 350 degrees. Place chicken skin side up in a baking dish. Mix mustard, butter, and tarragon and brush on chicken. Bake for about 1 hour or until golden. Season with salt and serve.

Serves 4

# Pesto Chicken

1 lb. chicken tenderloins

1/2 cup pesto (store-bought or recipe from page 134)

1 Tbsp. lemon juice

1-2 Tbsp. coconut oil or olive oil

Remove any moisture from the chicken with a paper towel. Coat the chicken with the oil. Combine the pesto with the lemon juice and rub all over the chicken. Place it on a broiler pan and broil 4 inches from the heat source for several minutes or until it just starts to brown. Turn over and cook the other side until it starts to brown. Alternately, it can be cooked on a grill. Season to taste with sea salt.

Serving suggestions: Serve as a main entrée topped with tomatoes marinated in a vinaigrette with chopped herbs. Or serve cut up in a green salad or a pasta salad. Serves 2-3

---

# Teriyaki Steak Kabobs

1/2 cup soy sauce or tamari sauce

1/4 cup apple cider vinegar

2 Tbsp. unrefined brown sugar (Rapadura brand, etc...)

2 Tbsp. chopped onion

1 Tbsp. mild oil, such as avocado oil, grapeseed, or olive oil

1 clove garlic, minced

1/2 tsp. ground ginger

1/8 tsp. pepper

2 lbs. boneless grass-fed beef sirloin steak

In a bowl, combine the first 8 ingredients. Trim the fat from the steak and slice across the grain into 1/2 inch strips. Place in a dish and let marinate for 20 minutes or up to 3 hours. Remove from marinade and thread meat onto skewers. Grill uncovered over medium-hot heat for 7-10 minutes or until meat reaches desired doneness, turning often. Serves 6

# Asian Garlic Salmon

1 lb. fresh salmon

2 tsp. lemon or lime juice

2 cloves garlic, minced

1 tsp honey

1 tsp freshly grated ginger

3 Tbsp. soy sauce

1 Tbsp coconut oil

Mix ingredients together except for the salmon.  Place the salmon in the marinade and marinate for 20 minutes or several hours. Place salmon on a baking sheet.  Drizzle melted coconut oil on salmon and cook in the oven at 350 until it flakes apart when a fork is inserted into the meat and twisted.  Or it can be cooked on the grill.   Serves 2

---

# Grilled Rosemary Mustard Chicken

3-4 lbs. chicken thighs

1/3 cup Dijon mustard

1/3 cup mayonnaise

1/2 tsp. chopped fresh rosemary

Sea salt and pepper

Heat a gas grill to medium high.  Mix the mustard with the mayonnaise and rosemary.  Season the chicken with salt and pepper, then coat it with the mustard mixture.  Place chicken on the grill and cook, turning once until done.  Serves 4-6

**Variations:** You can add other chopped herbs, pesto, or hot sauce to the mustard-mayonnaise mixture.

# Stir Fry

1-2 cups broccoli florets, chopped

1 zucchini, chopped

1 onion, chopped

1/2 red bell pepper, chopped

1 large carrot, thinly sliced

2 cups Bok choy or nappa cabbage, chopped

1 cup snow peas or sugar snap peas

2 garlic cloves, minced

1/4 tsp. ginger root, minced

2 Tbsp. soy sauce

1/2 tsp. sesame oil

3 Tbsp. olive oil

Cooked meat or seafood (optional)

Cooked rice

Heat large skillet over medium high heat for a couple minutes. Add the oil, broccoli and onion and cook for 2-3 minutes, then add the remaining vegetables. Let cook 8-10 minutes, stirring often. Add the minced garlic and ginger and cook for 1 minute. Add soy sauce and sesame oil. Turn down the heat and cover. Add cooked meat and serve over rice. Serves 2-3

## Veggie Tacos

1/4 cup sweet onion

7 sun-dried tomatoes

1/2 tsp. cumin

1/2 tsp. garlic powder

1 cup raw walnuts

Sea salt to taste

2 ripe avocados

1 Tbsp. fresh lemon or lime juice

5-6 medium size romaine lettuce leaves

Kefir sauce, optional, page 126

Cheese, shredded, optional

2 Tbsp. chopped cilantro

Cut the avocado into cubes and put into a bowl. Sprinkle with the citrus juice and some sea salt and mash with a fork.

Place the onion, sun-dried tomatoes, cumin, garlic powder and walnuts in a food processor and process until finely ground. Taste and adjust seasonings.

Place the avocado mixture down the middle of each lettuce leaf and top with the walnut/taco mixture.

Finish it off with the chopped cilantro, kefir sauce and shredded cheese, if desired.

Serves 3-4

# Cannelloni

**Tomato Sauce:**

>    7 sun-dried tomatoes, in oil or softened in water
>
>    1 tsp. fresh lemon juice
>
>    2 Tbsp. olive oil
>
>    1/2 tsp. garlic powder
>
>    2 tsp. fresh herbs, such as basil, thyme, or oregano
>
>    2 cups tomatoes, chopped
>
>    1/2 tsp. sea salt
>
>    2 dates

2 zucchini, chopped

1/2 tsp. nutmeg

1 cup raw cashews, soaked in water to soften

2 Tbsp. fresh lemon juice

1 tsp. sea salt or to taste

2-3 long, thin Chinese eggplant, peeled


Place all the tomato sauce ingredients in a food processor and mix until smooth. Taste and adjust seasonings. Set the sauce aside.

To make the filling, place the zucchini, nutmeg, cashews, lemon juice and salt in the food processor and process until well combined and smooth.

Using a mandolin or a vegetable peeler, shave long wide strips from the eggplant. This is the shell of the cannelloni. Place 4 strips on a plate, side by side, overlapping slightly, to make a square mat of eggplant. Place a few tablespoons of the filling along one edge and roll the up the eggplant to make a long tube. Top with the tomato sauce.

Repeat with the remaining eggplant strips and filling. You can garnish it with some pine nuts or freshly chopped herbs.

Serves 3-4

## Pizza

1 package Chebe bread mix, (or a gluten-free pizza crust)

2 eggs

2 Tbsp. olive oil

1/2 cup marinara sauce (see recipe on page 145) or storebought sauce

1/2 cup pesto (recipe on page 134 or storebought)

1 large sweet onion, sliced thinly

2 zucchini, sliced thinly

2 Tbsp. olive oil

Sea salt

1/4 cup grated Parmesan cheese, optional

15 slices of natural pepperoni, optional

Preheat oven to 350 degrees. Prepare chebe mix by placing the powdered mix in a bowl. Add 2 eggs and 2 Tbsp. olive oil and mix with a fork. Add 4-5 Tbsp. filtered water and mix in. Knead dough for a minute or so to combine.

Divide dough in half and roll out each piece onto a baking sheet into a round circle. Bake for 20 minutes.

While chebe is baking place the sliced zucchini and onions in a bowl and drizzle with the 2 Tbsp. olive oil. Stir gently to coat.

After Chebe is finished cooking, remove from oven and place each crust on a cooling rack. Spread the pesto on the crusts and top with the tomato sauce.

Place the zucchini and onion slices on the baking sheet in a single layer. Broil about 4 inches from the heating element until they start to get brown spots. Turn off broiler and leave in oven for another few minutes.

Remove from oven, season with salt, and place the cooked zucchini on the pizza crusts, top with the onions, grated cheese, and pepperoni if desired. Cut into quarters with a sharp knife or pizza cutter and serve immediately.   Makes 2 medium pizzas.

# Pumpkin Seed Pesto Pasta

1 1/2 cups raw pumpkin seeds, soaked in water for 1 hour or more

1/2 cup olive oil

2 cups parsley (or basil, spinach, or kale)

1 clove garlic

1 Tbsp. lemon juice

1/2 tsp. sea salt

4-5 yellow squash, peeled

Put all ingredients except the yellow squash into a food processor and process until coarsely ground.

Using a vegetable peeler, peel long, thin strips lengthwise down the squash, rotating as you peel. Stop when you reach the center seeds. Place in a bowl and sprinkle with sea salt and some olive oil. Stir gently to coat and serve with the pumpkin seed pesto over the squash noodles. Serves 4

# Chicken with Garlic and Roasted Red Peppers

4-5 chicken thighs, with skin on

3 jarred roasted red peppers, drained and cut into strips

1/4 cup chicken broth

1/4 tsp. garlic powder

3 cloves garlic, smashed

1/4 tsp. dried thyme

2 Tbsp. arrowroot powder

Place chicken in a large skillet and sprinkle each thigh with some of the garlic powder, thyme, and sea salt. Pour in the broth, and sprinkle the red pepper and garlic around chicken in pan.

Cook, covered, on lowest possible heat for 4-6 hours. Remove chicken and peppers from pan and place on a platter. Add the arrowroot to the broth and use a whisk to combine it well. Increase the heat to medium heat while stirring the broth until it becomes thick. Taste and add salt if needed. Serve sauce over the chicken. Serves 2-3.

# Fish with Fennel and Leeks

2-3 leeks, rinsed well and thinly sliced

1 fennel bulb, thinly sliced

2 fish fillets

2 Tbsp. coconut oil

Sea salt

Saute the leeks and fennel in some coconut oil until they are soft. Dry the fillets with paper towels, coat with coconut oil, and broil 4 inches from the heating element for 4-7 minutes, or until it just starts to flake when a fork is inserted in the meat. Add sea salt to taste.

To serve, place the leek mixture on a plate and top with the fish.

Serves 2

---

# Lentils

2 cups French green lentils, soaked overnight in water

3 cloves garlic

1/2 tsp. cumin

1 tsp. dried thyme

Pinch of red pepper flakes

Drain lentils and put in a pot. Add the garlic, cumin, red pepper flakes, and thyme. Add enough water to cover lentils by a half inch or so. Bring to a boil, reduce to a simmer and cook about 30-45 minutes or until done. Add 2 Tbsp. sea salt to the lentils and let sit to absorb the salt.

Serves 4

# Chicken Pesto Pasta

16 oz. gluten free pasta (bow tie, spirals, etc…)

1 1/2 cups fresh asparagus, cut into 1 inch pieces

1 1/4 cups sliced fresh mushrooms

1 red bell pepper, diced

2 tsp. minced garlic

2 Tbsp. olive oil

2 cups cooked chicken, cubed

1 can artichoke hearts (water packed), drained

1 cup Pesto (page 134)

1/2 cup sun-dried tomatoes, soaked in water 1 hour, drained and chopped

1 tsp. sea salt

1/8 tsp. crushed red pepper flakes

1 cup parmesan cheese (optional)

Cook pasta according to the package directions and add the asparagus during the last 3 minutes of cooking. Drain.

In a skillet, sauté the mushrooms, bell pepper, and garlic until tender.

Reduce the heat and stir in the chicken, artichokes, pesto, tomatoes, salt and pepper flakes. Cook 2-3 minutes longer or until heated through.

Drain pasta and toss with the chicken mixture. Sprinkle with cheese and nuts.

Serves 6-8

## Meatballs

1 1/2 lbs. ground meat (buffalo, beef, venison, turkey, etc..)

1/2 cup gluten free bread crumbs

1/2 tsp. garlic powder

1 Tbsp. Dijon mustard

2 Tbsp. fresh parsley minced

1 Tbsp. fresh basil, minced or 1 tsp. dried basil

1 egg, beaten

1/4 tsp. sea salt

1/8 tsp. cinnamon

1/8 tsp. nutmeg

Pinch of cayenne pepper

Mix all ingredients and form into walnut sized balls. Place on a rimmed baking sheet and bake at 350 for 25-30 minutes or until slightly browned and cooked through.     Serves 4-6

---

## Chicken with Onions and Mushrooms

4-5 chicken thighs, with the skin on

1/2 cup onion, cut into strips

4-6 ounces sliced mushrooms

2 garlic cloves

1/2 tsp. thyme

1 bay leaf

1/4 cup chicken broth

2 Tbsp. arrowroot powder

Place chicken in a large skillet and sprinkle each thigh with the thyme and sea salt. Pour in the broth in the pan, and sprinkle the garlic, onion, bay leaf, and mushrooms around the chicken in the pan.

Cook, covered, on lowest possible heat for 4-6 hours. Remove chicken, onions, and mushrooms from pan and place on a platter. Add the arrowroot to the broth in the pan and use a whisk to combine it well. Increase the heat to medium heat while stirring the broth until it becomes thick. Taste and add salt if needed. Serve sauce over the chicken with the onions and mushrooms.     Serves 2-3.

# Soups

# The Benefits of Broth

Due to modern meat processing techniques that offer boneless chicken breasts and individual fillets of fish, there has been a decline in using the bones to make broth. Now, people use canned broths or bouillion cubes which are loaded with neuro-toxic monosodium glutamate. But our grandmothers and ancestors knew the benefits of broth and made good use of the bones of animals and fish when they made it.

When they are properly prepared, meat broths are extremely nutritious because they contain minerals from the bone and cartilage in a form that is easy to assimilate. Broth also supplies gelatin. Gelatin attracts digestive juices to the surface of cooked foods and allows those foods to be digested easily. That is one reason why homemade chicken soup is so good for you when you are sick. And why foods cooked with gelatin-rich broth are so easily digested and nourishing.

---

## Chicken Broth

6-8 lbs. chicken parts (raw or cooked)

2 medium onions, halved

3 carrots, coarsely chopped

2 celery stalks, chopped

1 leek, rinsed well, and cut in large pieces (optional)

Herbs (optional):

> 1-2 Tbsp. dried thyme
>
> 1/2 bunch fresh parsley
>
> 8-10 peppercorns
>
> 3 bay leaves

Place all ingredients into a stockpot and add enough cold filtered water to cover everything by about 1-2 inches. Bring to a boil, then reduce heat to a slow simmer, skimming off the scum that appears on the top of the broth with a spoon. Let simmer for 3-8 hours.

Remove from heat and strain broth. Pour into containers, label, and store in the refrigerator or freezer. It will keep for 4-5 days in the refrigerator (bring it to a boil for 10 minutes and it can be stored for 5 more days), and it will keep frozen for many months.

## Cream of Vegetable Soup

1 cup onion, chopped

2 cloves garlic, optional

2 Tbsp. butter or olive oil

Herbs: 1 tsp. thyme, bay leaf, basil, or other herbs

3 cups chicken stock

2 cups of one vegetable, such as broccoli, cauliflower, etc..

Sea salt to taste

1/2 cup almond milk

Saute the onion in the oil or butter until it softens over medium heat. Add the garlic and sauté for a minute. Add the herbs, vegetable, and broth and bring to a boil. Cover, reduce heat, and simmer for 20-25 minutes or until the vegetable is tender when pierced with a fork. Puree with a stick blender. Add cream and season to taste. Serves 2-3

---

## Chicken Soup

2 Tbsp. coconut oil or olive oil

2 leeks, thinly sliced

2 carrots, thinly sliced

1/2 cup sliced mushrooms

2 1/2 cups chicken broth

1 cup cooked chicken (from making broth), chopped

1 cup frozen green peas

1 Tbsp. chopped fresh parsley

1/2 tsp. fresh lemon juice

1/2 cup gluten-free pasta (optional)

Heat oil in a large saucepan over medium heat. Add the leeks and carrots and cook for 5 minutes, stirring often. Add the mushrooms and cook for 2-3 more minutes. Pour in the broth, peas, pasta, lemon juice, and bring to a boil. Reduce heat, and simmer for 15-20 minutes or until vegetables are tender. Add cooked chicken and season to taste.

Serves 2

## Carrot Soup

3 cups freshly made carrot juice

1 small avocado

4 Tbsp. thick coconut cream

1 tsp. lime juice (optional)

1 Tbsp. minced ginger root

1/4 tsp. sea salt

A touch of agave or stevia if needed for sweetness

Blend all ingredients until smooth in a blender. Taste and adjust seasonings. Serve cool or at room temperature.

Serves 2-3

---

## Split Pea Soup

1 lb. dry split peas

8 cups chicken broth

2 medium potatoes, cubed

2 large onions, chopped

2 carrots, chopped

1/2 cup celery, chopped

1 tsp. marjoram

1 tsp. poultry seasoning

1 tsp. rubbed sage

1/2 tsp. pepper

1/2 tsp. basil

1/2 tsp. sea salt

Combine all ingredients in a large soup pot and bring to a boil. Reduce heat, cover and simmer for 1 1/4 to 1 1/2 hours or until vegetables are tender.

Serves 12

# Italian Vegetable Soup

3 Tbsp. olive oil

1 large onion, chopped

2 celery ribs, sliced

6 carrots, sliced

4 cloves garlic, minced

2 16 oz. cans diced tomatoes

1 28 oz. can crushed tomatoes

12 cups chicken broth

2 cups cooked garbanzo beans

2 cups cooked kidney beans

2 bay leaves

2 medium zucchini, diced

2 summer squash, diced

1/2 cup frozen peas

1/2 bunch basil leaves, chopped

2 tsp. balsamic vinegar

Sea salt to taste


In a large pot, sauté the onion, celery, and carrots over medium heat for 5-8 minutes. Add garlic and cook one more minute. Add the tomatoes, broth, beans, herbs, squash, and cook for 30 minutes. Add the peas, basil, vinegar and cook 2 more minutes. Season to taste and remove the bay leaves before serving.

Serves 10-12

## Avocado Soup

1 small zucchini

1 ripe avocado

1 cup filtered water

1/4 cup sweet, mild onion

1/2 a lime, juiced

Zest of 1/4 of the lime

1/4 tsp. cumin

A pinch of cayenne pepper, or to taste

1 tsp. sea salt

3 stems of fresh cilantro

### Salsa for topping the soup:

1/4 cup mango, diced

1/4 cup tomato or red bell pepper, diced

1/8 cup sweet onion, diced

1 Tbsp. fresh cilantro, chopped

Put all soup ingredients (not the Salsa ingredients) into a high speed blender and blend until smooth. Add water to thin to desired consistency if necessary.

Mix salsa ingredients together in a small bowl. Place 2 tablespoons of salsa on top of soup in the serving bowl.

Serves 1-2

# Spicy Bean Soup

1 onion, chopped

2 carrots, chopped

1 clove of garlic, minced

2 Tbsp. olive oil

1/2 tsp. cumin

A pinch of red pepper flakes

3 cups of chicken broth

2 cups cooked beans, pinto or black beans

In a large pot, sauté the onion and carrots over medium heat for 5-8 minutes. Add garlic and cook one more minute. Add the broth, beans, cumin, and red pepper flakes. Bring to a boil, reduce to a simmer and let cook for 15-20 minutes.

Puree soup with a hand-blender. Garnish with chopped cilantro and serve.

Serves 2-4

## Pumpkin Soup

1 1/2 Tbsp. coconut oil

1/2 onion, chopped

3/4 cup carrot, chopped

1 garlic clove, minced

1 bay leaf

1 whole clove

4-5 cups chicken broth

1 small pie pumpkin, peeled, seeded, and chopped

1/2 tsp. ground nutmeg

1/2 tsp. ground cinnamon

1/4 tsp. allspice

5-6 drops stevia extract or 1 Tbsp. honey

1 tsp. sea salt

1 cup coconut milk

Melt coconut oil in a large pot over medium heat. Add the carrot and onion and cook until they get soft, about 8-10 minutes. Add the garlic and cook another minute. Add broth, bay leaf, clove, pumpkin, nutmeg, cinnamon, and allspice. Cook 20-30 minutes, or until pumpkin is cooked through. Add stevia and coconut milk. Puree soup with a stick blender and add sea salt to taste. Taste and adjust seasonings.

Serves 4

# Creamy Tomato Soup

2-3 cups raw ripe tomatoes

1 cup raw macadamias

1/2 cup sun-dried tomatoes

2 Tbsp. tamari

1/2 jalapeno pepper or chipotle pepper (to taste)

Filtered water

Place all ingredients into a high speed blender and blend until smooth and creamy. Add water to thin if necessary. Taste and adjust seasonings.

Serves 3-4

## Lentil Soup

1 cup carrots, finely chopped

1 cup onion, finely chopped

1/2 cup celery, finely chopped

1 cup leeks, finely chopped

2 cups lentils (preferably soaked in water overnight and drained)

10 cups chicken broth (or part broth and part water)

2 garlic cloves, minced

2 bay leaves

1/2 tsp. dried thyme

1 Tbsp. fresh chopped parsley

In a large soup pot, sauté the carrots, onion, celery, and leeks in a few tablespoons of olive oil until they start to soften. Add the lentils, stock, garlic, bay leaves, thyme, and parsley. Bring to a boil, reduce heat, and simmer for 30 minutes. Season to taste with sea salt.

This soup freezes well.

## Garlic Beef Soup

1 lb. beef, buffalo, or venison steak, cut into small strips

2 Tbsp. butter or olive oil

1/2 onion, chopped

4 cloves garlic, minced

1 carrot, sliced

1-2 cups mixed chopped vegetables, such as bok choy, napa cabbage, broccoli, red bell pepper, kale, etc..

2 cups beef or chicken broth

2 Tbsp. soy sauce

Saute meat in oil, then remove from pan. Cook onion, carrot, and garlic in pan until they start to soften. Add broth, vegetables, and soy sauce. Bring to a boil, reduce heat, and simmer for 15-20 minutes. Add meat to the soup and serve. Serves 1-2

# Vegetable Chili (Raw)

1 portabello mushroom, finely chopped

1/2 cup chopped red or green onion, optional

1 red bell pepper, finely chopped

1/2 cup chopped carrots

1 cup sun-dried tomatoes, soaked in water 1 hour

2 cups water, fresh, or from the soaked tomatoes

1 Tbsp. olive oil

1/2 tsp. garlic powder

1/2 Tbsp. dried basil or oregano

1 tsp. chili powder

1-2 tsp. cumin

1/2 Tbsp. apple cider vinegar

1 Tbsp. agave or honey

1/4 tsp. cayenne pepper or to taste

1 cup frozen corn, thawed

Sea salt to taste

Place the mushrooms in a large bowl. Place the pepper, onion, and carrot in the food processor and process until finely chopped. Blend remaining ingredients, except for the corn, together in a blender until smooth. Add to the vegetables in the bowl, mix in the corn, and transfer to a saucepan. Warm gently on the stove on low heat, stirring often. Do not cook at a high temperature. This is meant to be a raw soup.

Serves 2

# Notes

# Desserts

# Cobbler

## Topping:

3/4 cup raw almonds, ground in a food processor to a fine meal

3/4 cup arrowroot powder

6 Tbsp. coconut oil

1/4 cup unrefined sugar (such as Rapadura, etc..)

1/4 tsp. sea salt

1 tsp. vanilla extract

## Filling:

4 very ripe pears or peaches, 3 sliced thin, and 1 chopped

1/2 cup raisins, soaked in water to soften (optional)

1 Tbsp. cinnamon

1/2 Tbsp. fresh lemon juice

1/2 tsp. sea salt

In a greased pie plate or other serving dish, place the sliced pears. Place the topping ingredients in a food processor and mix until it just starts to clump together. Do not overmix or it will become creamy like nut butter. It should still look crumbly. Place it in a bowl.

Next, place the chopped pear or peach in the food processor with the raisins, cinnamon, lemon juice and salt. Blend until smooth. Pour this sauce over the sliced pears in the pie plate and mix to coat all the pears. Crumble the topping over the pear mixture and serve. It can also be served warmed slightly, but this is a raw dish and is not meant to be cooked in the oven.

Serves 4-6

Note: This recipe works well for any soft, ripe fruit. You can also add some berries with the other fruit. Blueberry and Peach is a nice combination. The raisins do not have to be soaked, but they blend easier if they are softened.

# Brownie Bars

1 1/2 cups raw almonds, ground finely in the food processor

6 Tbsp. carob or cacao powder

6 Tbsp. coconut oil

2-3 tsp. honey or agave

2 tsp. vanilla extract

Pinch of sea salt

A big pinch of cinnamon

Sesame seeds for topping or Fudge Topping

Mix all ingredients in a bowl and press into a small oiled dish. Sprinkle with the sesame seeds or top with the Fudge Topping recipe below. Chill in the refrigerator until firm. Cut into bars and store in refrigerator.

# Fudge Topping

1 cup soft coconut oil or butter

1 cup raw honey or agave

1 cup raw cacao powder or carob powder

1 tsp. vanilla extract

1/2 tsp. sea salt

Combine all ingredients in a bowl and mix well.

Note: This also makes a nice icing for cakes or cupcakes.

## Chocolate Ice Cream

4 Tbsp. raw chocolate powder

14-16 medjool dates, pit removed

4 Tbsp. raw nut butter or coconut butter

1 Tbsp. vanilla extract

Pinch of cinnamon

Pinch of sea salt

2 1/2 cups filtered water

Place all ingredients and only a small amount of the water in a food processor and mix until smooth.  Once it is smooth, add the remaining water and mix.  Freeze in an ice cream maker.

## Almond Joy

1 cup coconut oil

1/4 cup honey or agave

1/4 cup almond butter

Dash of salt

1 tsp. vanilla extract

1/4 cup raw chocolate powder

1/4 cup sliced or chopped almonds

Place coconut oil in a saucepan and melt over low heat.  Combine remaining ingredients and stir until well blended.  Pour into a small serving dish and place in the refrigerator to chill until solid.  Cut into bars.  Store in the refrigerator.

## Strawberry Cheesecake

For the crust, use the recipe on page 176

**Filling:**

2 cups fresh strawberries

1 cup cashews

1 ounce coconut butter or cacao butter

2 tsp. vanilla extract

1/4 cup raw honey or agave

1 Tbsp. fresh lemon juice

1/4 tsp. sea salt

Place all ingredients in a high speed blender or a food processor and process until smooth and creamy. Pour filling into the crust and let chill in the refrigerator until it thickens.

Note: Soaking the cashews for an hour in water and draining them before blending makes it easier to blend them into a creamy consistency.

---

## Chocolate Pudding

2 ripe avocados

3/4 cup  agave nectar or honey

1/2-3/4 cup raw chocolate powder or carob powder

2 Tbsp. coconut butter

1 Tbsp. vanilla extract

Dash of sea salt

Dash of cinnamon

Place all ingredients in a food processor and mix until smooth. Taste and adjust seasonings to your liking. You can add more chocolate powder for a richer, dark chocolate flavor.

# Pie Crusts and Fillings

## Easy Pie Crust

2 cups raw almonds or other nuts

1/2 cup dates or other dried fruit

A big pinch of sea salt

In a food processor, grind the almonds until finely ground. Add the dates or dried fruit and salt and grind until it starts to clump together and form a ball. A small amount of water may be necessary if it does not clump together. Press this into the sides and the bottom of a pie plate. Makes 1 pie crust.

---

## Pie Fillings

### Blueberry filling:

5 cups blueberries

2 bananas

1 1/2 Tbsp. raw honey, agave, or stevia

1/2 tsp. vanilla extract

In a food processor, combine 4 cups of the blueberries, the bananas, and the remaining ingredients. Blend until smooth. Remove from the food processor and stir the remaining berries. Pour into crust. Refrigerate at least 3 hours so it can firm up.

---

### Mango filling:

4 ripe mangos

6 bananas

Peel the mangos and cut meat off the seed and place in food processor with 4 of the bananas. Blend until smooth. Slice the remaining bananas and place in a bowl. Add the mango mixture and stir well. Pour into the pie crust and refrigerate a few hours.

## Apple filling:

7 apples

8 dates or 1/2 cup dried fruit, soaked in water for an hour

1/2 cup raisins

1/2 lemon, juiced

1 tsp. cinnamon

In a food processor, blend 2 apples with the dates until smooth. Pour into a bowl and set aside. Next, place 4 apples in the processor and pulse chop into tiny pieces. Combine them with the date mixture and add the cinnamon, lemon juice, and raisins. Mix well and pour into pie crust. Let stand in refrigerator for about an hour.

## Strawberry filling:

2 cups cashews, soaked 1-2 hours or 1 1/2 cups nut butter

1/4 cup lemon juice

1/4 cup agave

5 drops stevia extract

1/2 cup fresh or frozen strawberries

3/4 cup coconut oil or 1/2 cup coconut butter

1/2 cup water

1 Tbsp. vanilla extract

1/2 tsp. nutritional yeast, optional

1/2 tsp. sea salt

1 cup fresh strawberries for topping the pie, sliced

Blend all ingredients except for the extra 1 cup of strawberries for topping in a high speed blender until very smooth. Pour a small amount of filling into the bottom of the crust. Place half of the sliced strawberries over the filling, then pour the remaining filling into the crust. Chill in freezer 1-2 hours or place in refrigerator overnight. Top with remaining sliced strawberries just before serving.

## Chocolate filling:

1 1/2 cups raw cashews, soaked in water for 1 hour and drained

1/2 cup water

1/2 cup agave or honey

1/2 cup coconut oil, melted on low heat

1/2 tsp. vanilla extract

1/4 tsp. sea salt

1 cup raw chocolate powder

Blend all ingredients together until very smooth.  Pour into crust and chill overnight in refrigerator.

---

*This makes a very decadant pie!*

## Chocolate Peanut Butter Pie filling:

1 cup peanut butter or any other nut butter

Chocolate Filling or the Chocolate pudding recipe

1 pie crust

Layer the bottom of the pie crust with peanut butter or nut butter.  Then spread the above chocolate filling on top of the nut butter.  Refrigerate or serve immediately.

Makes 1 pie.

# Pumpkin Pie

3 cups raw butternut squash, peeled and chopped

1/4 cup agave

2 Tbsp. maple syrup or 4 medjool dates

1/4 cup coconut butter or coconut cream

1/4 cup raw cashews or raw cashew butter

1 tsp. cinnamon

1/4 tsp. nutmeg

1/4 tsp. ginger

Pinch of cloves

1 pie crust (see recipe on previous page)

Place all ingredients, except the crust, into a food processor and process until smooth. Pour into the pie crust and refrigerate for a couple of hours before serving. Makes 1 pie.

---

# Date Candies

6 medjool dates, with pit removed

1/2 tsp. vanilla extract

6 tsp. coconut butter

6 raw macadamia nuts or raw almonds

Open up each date and place several drops of vanilla extract inside. Then place a tsp of the coconut butter and a nut in each one. Squeeze slightly to close. Makes 6

# Gingered Fruit

1 cup dried or fresh figs

1/3 cup fresh lime juice

1/4 cup raw honey or agave

2 tsp. finely grated fresh ginger root

2 red grapefruits, sectioned

2 ripe pears, cored and diced

1 bunch grapes

If you are using dried figs, let them rehydrate in warm water for 20 minutes.  Cut figs in half.

Mix together the lime juice, honey and ginger  and toss with all of the fruit in a bowl.  Let marinate for 30-60 minutes before serving.

Note:  This makes a great topping for yogurt.

---

# Caramel Apple Dip

8 Tbsp. nut butter (almond butter, cashew butter, etc...)

1 Tbsp. vanilla extract

4 medjool dates, pitted and chopped

1/2 tsp. cinnamon

Pinch of sea salt

2-3 Tbsp. water

1 Tbsp. agave

Fruit for dipping, such as apple slices

In a food processor, mix all the ingredients except the fruit in a food processor or blender until smooth.  Add water to thin if necessary.  Serve with fruit.

# Apple Spice Crumble Cake

## Filling:

       8 apples, peeled, cored, and thinly sliced

       1/4 cup dates, pitted

       1/4 cup raisins

       1/2 Tbsp. lemon juice

       1 tsp. cinnamon

       1 thin slice of fresh ginger root

2 cups almonds or other nuts

3/4 cup dates, pitted or raisins

1/2 cup arrowroot powder

2 Tbsp. coconut oil

3 tsp. cinnamon

1/4 tsp. sea salt

1/2 tsp. dried ginger

In a food processor, place 2 of the apples along with the other filling ingredients and process until smooth. In a large bowl, mix the filling with the remaining sliced apples.

Put the nuts in a food processor and process until it is as fine as possible. Add the dates and the rest of the ingredients and pulse until it is a crumbly mixture.

To assemble, press 1/3rd of the crumbled mixture into a 8 inch baking dish or pie plate. Layer 1/2 of the apple mixture on top and press down firmly. Sprinkle another 1/3rd of the crumble on top of the apples, followed by the remaining apple mixture. Press down and top with the rest of the crumble.

Serves 6

## Raw Chocolate Cups

1 cup coconut oil

1 cup raw almond butter

1 cup raw cacao powder

1 Tbsp. vanilla extract

1/2 cup agave nectar or raw honey

Pinch of sea salt

Place all ingredients in a food processor. Mix for 2-3 minutes. It will go from a thick, pudding-like consistency to a more liquid consistency. Taste and add more raw cacao or agave if necessary.

Put tiny paper liners into small muffin tins. Use a large syringe to pour the liquid chocolate into the paper cups. Fill the paper cups with the chocolate and place in the refrigerator to harden. Move to another airtight container and store in the refrigerator or freezer.

**Variations:** These can also be made with fillings, such as peanut butter, almond butter, slivered almonds, raspberries, coconut, etc...

### Nut Butter Cups

Place only a tiny bit of the chocolate liquid in each paper liner, so that they are only 1/4 full. Using a teaspoon, put a dollop of nut butter on top of the chocolate, then pour the remaining chocolate on top of the nut butter so it is completely covered.   Refrigerate until firm.

# Mango Berry Parfait

Mango Mousse:

       3 mangos, peeled and cut off the seed

       4 Tbsp. coconut butter or cream

       1 tsp. vanilla extract

       2 Tbsp. lime juice

       1 Tbsp. lime zest

       2-4 Tbsp. agave nectar or honey

       Pinch of salt

1 cup mixed berries

1 cup raw nuts

4 dates or other dried fruit

3 Tbsp. ground flax seeds

1/4 tsp. sea salt

1/2 tsp. cinnamon

Blend mango mousse ingredients until smooth. Place the raw nuts in a food processor and process to a fine meal. Add the dried fruit, flaxseeds, salt, and cinnamon and mix well.

In a parfait glass or wine glass, place a couple tablespoons of the nut mixture, layer it with some of the mango mousse, then the berries. Repeat layers and top with berries.

**Variation:** The Mango Mousse can be made into ice cream. Place frozen mango and the other ingredients in a food processor and mix until smooth for a soft-serve ice cream. Or you can use an ice-cream maker.

## Chocolate Chip Cookies

2 cups almond flour

1/4 tsp. sea salt

1/4 tsp. baking soda

10 Tbsp. coconut oil, melted

1 Tbsp. vanilla extract

1/2 cup agave or honey (or 2 Tbsp. agave and 8 drops stevia extract)

1 cup gluten-free chocolate chips

Mix all ingredients, except for the chocolate chips.  Add chocolate chips to dough and form into 1 inch balls.  Press balls slightly to flatten into a cookie shape and place on a parchment paper lined baking sheet.  Bake at 350 for 7-10 minutes, or until just starting to brown.

---

## Carrot Cake

1 cup whole grain, gluten-free flour

1 tsp. baking powder

1 tsp. baking soda

1 tsp. cinnamon

1/4 tsp. sea salt

2 eggs, beaten

1 cup packed grated carrots

4 oz. crushed pineapple

1/2 cup raisins

1/3 cup agave

1/4 cup coconut oil

Preheat the oven to 350 degrees.  Lightly oil a square baking dish.  In a large bowl, whisk the dry ingredients together until combined.  In another bowl, stir together the eggs, carrot, pineapple, raisins, sweetener, and oil.  Slowly add the wet ingredients to the dry until barely combined.  Pour into the dish and bake for 30-35 minutes, or until done.

# Cinnamon Pecan Macaroons

2 cups dried coconut (finely shredded and unsweetened)

1/2 cup almonds

1/2 cup coconut oil

1/4 cup maple syrup

1/4 cup agave

1 vanilla bean, scraped or 2 tsp. vanilla extract

1 heaping teaspoon cinnamon

1/2 cup chopped pecans

Pinch of sea salt

Place the almonds in a food processor and process until it is a flour or coarse meal, about 1 minute. Add the rest of the ingredients, except the pecans and mix until it starts to clump together. Add in the pecans and pulse a few times to chop them.

Using a cookie scoop, scoop the dough and place onto dehydrator trays. Dehydrate at 100 degrees 12-24 hours, depending on the size of your macaroon and your desired texture.

Makes about 2 dozen macaroons.

## Variation: Cranberry Cherry Macaroons

Add 1/4 cup dried cranberries and 1/4 cup dried chopped cherries to the above recipe. Omit the cinnamon and pecans.

# Notes

# Appendix:   Product Resources

**Agave Nectar**   Xagave is my favorite raw brand. (www.xagave.com)

**Almond Milk**   Almond Breeze is a good storebought alternative if you do not want to make it yourself.  Be sure to buy the unsweetened version.

**Breads (Gluten-free)**   Chebe bread mix (www.chebe.com), Udi's (www.udisglutenfree.com), and Rudi's are some of the better ones.

**Coconut Butter**   Artisana makes a delicious coconut butter that can be used in many ways (www.artisanafoods.com)

**Coconut Oil**   Coconut oil should be cold-pressed and have a slight coconut flavor.  Nutiva (www.nutiva.com) and Artisana (www.artisanafoods.com) and Wilderness Family Naturals (www.wildernessfamilynaturals.com)

**Cashew Butter, Raw and other Nut Butters**   Artisana makes the best! (www.artisanafoods.com)

**Fermented Vegetables**   Bubbies brand of dill pickles are made the old fashioned way through fermentation.  Also see www.rejuvenative.com.

**Flours, gluten free and whole grain**   Bob's Red Mill (www.bobsredmill.com) carries whole grain flour and gluten-free oats.

**Honey, raw**   Honey Gardens (www.honeygardens.com) or check your area for local beekeepers who sell raw, local honey.

**Olive Oil**   Olave is a very nice, low acidity , cold-pressed olive oil (www.olave.cl)

**Pasta**   For gluten free pasta, try Tinkyada brand (www.tinkyada.com)

**Produce**   Fresh fruits and vegetables are worth seeking out.  Local farmer's markets and community-supported-agriculture (CSA's) are popping up everywhere (www.localharvest.org)

**Sea Salt**   (www.celtic-seasalt.com)

**Stevia**   Most stevia has a strange aftertaste, but not the one from Body Ecology (www.bodyecology.com)

**Vanilla Extract**   The best vanilla extract is made by Nielsen Massey (www.nielsenmassey.com)

# Recommended Reading

*Nutrition and Physical Degeneration* by Weston A. Price: The nutrition classic of isolated people eating native diets and the effects of processed foods on human health. Everyone should read this book.

*Nourishing Traditions: The Cookbook That Challenges Politically Correct Nutrition and the Diet Dictocrats* by Sally Fallon: An excellent cookbook and resource for the practical application of Dr. Price's research to our modern diets.

*Eating in the Raw* and *The Raw 50* by Carol Alt: Supermodel Carol Alt has maintained a raw foods diet for over 10 years and her books have great information as well as delicious recipes.

*Wild Fermentation* by Sandor Katz: This book was one of the most helpful for learning the art of fermentation. His dill pickle recipe is amazingly easy and delicious!

*Living on Live Food* by Alissa Cohen: an excellent resource for easy raw vegan recipes and implementation of a raw food diet.

*The Raw Food Detox Diet* by Natalia Rose: One of the best books to explain how to transition to a more raw food diet. Includes some recipes.

*Food Healing for Man, The Nutrition Handbook*, and other books by Bernard Jensen: great information from a nutritional pioneer.

*The Maker's Diet* by Jordan Rubin: A lot of great information and some recipes.

*Simply Sugar and Gluten Free* by Amy Green: A wonderful cookbook of tasty gluten-free recipes.

*Omnivore's Dilemma* and other books by Michael Pollan: Excellent books on the problems with the modern food system.

*Living Raw Food* by Sarma Melngailis: A traditional chef turned onto raw foods provides a wealth of amazing recipes from her raw restaurant in New York, Pure Food and Wine.

*Food is Your Best Medicine* by Henry Bieler, M.D. How food can heal the body.

# Recommended Videos

*Food, Inc.*

*Food Matters*

*Fat, Sick, and Nearly Dead*

# Index

## About the Author

Becky Mauldin is a Naturopath and the owner of Pure Vitality, a business that helps to transform people's health.  She has authored the book, *Recipes for Life: A Raw Food Cookbook*, and has contributed articles to *Wise Traditions*, a journal of the Weston A. Price Foundation.

Having recovered from an incurable illness, she has learned firsthand how to attain optimal health.  She is passionate about helping others realize their potential for better health and vitality.  Her step-by-step health transforming system empowers people to transform their health easily and sustainably.

Prior to working as a Naturopath, Becky worked for many years as an artist and graphic designer.  In keeping with her passion for natural living, she and her husband hand-crafted their own log home, in which they currently reside in Douglasville, Georgia.

## Hungry for More?

Visit our website for even more recipes and resources on natural living and detoxification: www.getpurevitality.com

# Notes

# Notes

# Notes